The
ROAD MAP to
FERTILITY

A comprehensive guide to fertility for men and women

Dr David Greening

ROCKPOOL
PUBLISHING

A Rockpool book
PO Box 252
Summer Hill
NSW 2130
Australia

www.rockpoolpublishing.com.au
www.facebook.com/RockpoolPublishing
ISBN 978-1-925682-17-5

First published in 2018
Copyright text © David Greening, 2018
This edition published in 2018

A catalogue record for this
book is available from the
National Library of Australia

Cover design by Jessica Le, Rockpool Publishing
Editing and index by Lisa Macken
Images by Shutterstock except on pages xii, xiv, 12, 44, 78, 90, 100, 114, 134,
170, 206, 210, 226, 230 and 234 by Talman Madsen, www.talmanmadsen.com
Internal design and typesetting by Envisage Information Technology

Printed and bound in China

10 9 8 7 6 5 4 3 2 1

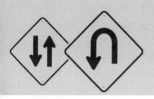 # About the author

David was born in New Zealand and studied medicine at Otago University in Dunedin. After a period of surgical training he changed to obstetrics and gynaecology. Taking a break from obstetrics and gynaecology training, he moved to Australia. Exciting work followed on Thursday Island in the remote Torres Strait then an appointment to the Royal Flying Doctor Service in Broken Hill, New South Wales.

A further year was spent with the Asian Emergency Assistance based in Singapore before he moved to Melbourne to recommence his specialist training at Monash Medical Centre.

In 2000 David began training in the sub-specialty of reproductive endocrinology and infertility, in Dublin, then at the prestigious IVF Hammersmith in London. In 2002 David moved back to Australia, joining Sydney IVF and subsequently started a practice in Wollongong. Along the way he completed a Masters in Bioethics at Monash University.

In 2015 he joined IVF Australia and, keeping with his belief that IVF should be affordable and accessible, started the Fertility Centre TFC Wollongong, one of the few low-cost IVF units in Australia.

He continues to live and work in Wollongong on the south coast of New South Wales and still practices obstetrics, delivering many of the babies of those couples he treated. David is married to Sian and has four children.

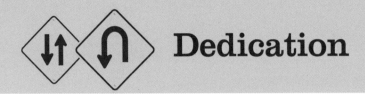 # Dedication

To Sian, who patiently travelled with me on the long road that *The Road Map to Fertility* became.

And to those many patients over the many years I had the privilege to help and to whom I gave directions

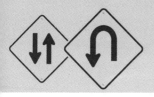 # One patient's story

My wife Sue and I had the great pleasure of meeting Dr David Greening while he was a member of the Sydney IVF team at Liverpool, New South Wales in 2002.

Before that, we had been through ten years of IVF hell – thirty-two attempts, several doctors and clinics, and a seemingly endless run of tests, cycles and failures.

My wife is a 5-foot tough nut and had to go through all of this. I was just the chauffeur, the person who had to 'fill up the cup' and try to support her when it didn't work – again, and again, and again!

Did any doctor do tests on me, ask me how I felt, or talk to me regularly? No! No support for men.

Thanks to Dr Greening we now have a daughter, born in 2003, and a son born in 2005.

The irony is, neither of our kids is the result of IVF.

The difference was Dr Greening. He said, 'Hang on, this isn't right. Something else is happening. We need to do some tests.' And so, he did. Finally, we were treated like human beings, spoken with and asked questions.

David had this new idea about improving my sperm DNA damage by more frequent ejaculation. After a little bit of uncomplicated testing and a simple treatment, we now have two kids. Dr Greening was also gracious enough to visit my wife in hospital and attend my daughter's christening.

My point is, guys, don't just go with the flow. Don't give up. Ask questions – you have a right.

Most of all, support your wife!

Read this book. It will help.

Gary

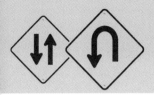 # You are not alone

Fertility is something that men assume they have. From the time they develop their first sexual feelings they assume they will be fertile men. Everywhere they look there are couples with children – on the TV, in books and magazines and in their social circle.

In fact, fertility cannot be assumed and is not as straightforward as many men believe. When infertility arrives on the scene it can be a rude shock. It turns up in as many as one in six couples and that number rises in older couples. It sometimes sneaks up slowly over time as a couple tries to conceive without success. Around them, their friends, colleagues and strangers seem to do it easily. Sometimes it arrives without warning, like a car crash, because of illness or injury. Sometimes, due to a congenital problem, infertility has been in the background from birth. Often infertility is self-inflicted through lifestyle or is the result of an acquired illness. And then there are the difficult instances of unexplained infertility, where answers elude the doctors.

Men have often been sidelined in the assessment of fertility as the female partner gets the most attention. Yet it is infertile men who are actually the problem in up to one third of infertile couples and in fact are the number one factor in infertility. It is called the 'male factor'. For men this can come as a surprise and, almost always, a huge shock. They assume they're men, and men are fertile, right? Real men are fertile, aren't they?

'Hey! If I'm the cause I'm not a real man!'

To many men this can be very confronting – egos are shattered, confidence is literally crushed.

If fertility is like a road trip then historically men have been passengers, tending to sit in the back seat. For thousands of years fertility has been seen as being women's business – the mysterious ability to conceive and nurture a small human through to childbirth was not man's domain. Today, so many of the questions about fertility have been answered and the male part is well understood, yet when couples have a standard consultation with a medical professional, in most cases the female partner drives the conversation. Most of the literature written is directed at the female partner.

I want this book to help men climb into the front seat and get involved. Don't sit in the back seat: join your partner in the front and form a team.

Think of it as a road trip. Before you leave, you plan, determining the route and assembling the required equipment. You try to cover all eventualities – you get the car serviced and check the trailer. You make sure all is in place before you leave the driveway.

The same applies to fertility: there are things to plan. When you start the drive (towards fertility) the route may not be straightforward, as things can arise on your journey towards a pregnancy and a child.

I am going to stick to this road map analogy throughout this book. There will be chapters on planning the fertility trip and chapters on driving to that destination, chapters about you and chapters about your partner.

What we know now about fertility and infertility makes it a good time to be alive. Much more is known now, and the issue is on the agenda for good. I have included information about female fertility as well.

Same-sex men and women and single people can conceive a child with modern medicine, through such technologies as IVF with donor eggs, a surrogate or the use of donor sperm. Fertility treatments may apply to people in different ways.

Author John Gray, in *Men are from Mars, Women are from Venus,* said that men want to fix things. It is in our nature. We love to work with cars and tinker under the bonnet. We plan our fishing trips down to the smallest detail. We like to know the rules – how a game of rugby works, or ice hockey, or soccer.

But sometimes we are not very good at reading instructions because we like to think we just know how something works. Remember the old saying, 'When in doubt, read the instructions'?

When confronted with the problem, frustrations and disappointments can be acute. Infertility is a silent, almost hidden epidemic and most men are not experts on fertility. Look around you at the shopping centre. Count six couples: one of those couples is having trouble conceiving. It is not a small number – the incidence of infertility is higher than most other sicknesses.

This book is designed to be instructional – a guidebook for both men and women to help them learn about their fertility. It can be read in two ways – before you have a problem (to understand fertility and the way things work), or when you have a problem (to gain some insights and possible solutions for the problem).

We all want to win – it's in our nature. Fertility is a sort of race that we all want to win, to arrive at the destination of parenthood and do our small part to contribute to the human race. Like the coach says, preparation aids performance. If we put in the preparation we will perform better.

This book will teach you what is under your bonnet and how it runs, what can go wrong and what to do to fix it.

This is not a medical textbook for doctors; it is written as much as possible in plain English. Occasionally there will be some medical jargon that will be explained, but the purpose of this book is to inform you and arm you with the knowledge you will need to get a grip on this topic. It is a road map to follow. You can find all sorts of information in here and skip ahead at any time.

Start your engines and drive on!

David Greening

MB, ChB, FRACGP, MBioeth, FRANZCOG, CREI

www.davidgreening.com.au

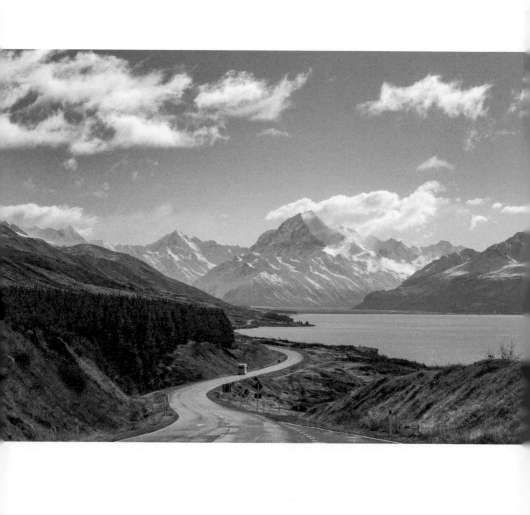

Contents

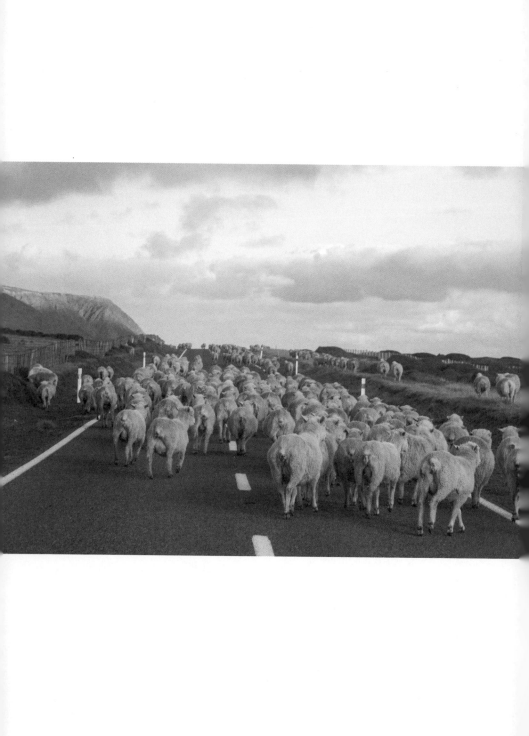

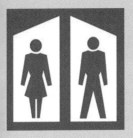

CHAPTER 1

The basics of conception

In the minds of many men, just being male should be enough. For many, the assumption is that real men can father a child. But sometimes that isn't the case. You might be an amazing specimen of manhood, with defined muscles, a jaw as square as a right angle, tall and handsome, but if you have a fertility problem that self-perception can crumble. I have seen it many times.

One of my patients ticked every box and had an abundance of self-confidence that literally oozed out of him. When he and his partner returned for their second visit I went over their results. His partner was fine – there were no obvious problems with her fertility. However, he had a very low sperm count of about one to two million (around forty million is considered 'fertile'). When I told him, he slumped forward and couldn't speak for several minutes – elbows on knees, head down processing this news. His ego was like a balloon that had popped.

Men see themselves as fathers, outside playing with a son or daughter, reading to their children at night, passing on their wisdom, providing for their children and watching them grow up. They expect to be grandparents one day. To be denied this is one of the toughest situations men and their partners will ever find themselves in.

I fortunately sorted this couple out with IVF. It worked well, and they have a family now.

Before we look at the basics of male fertility, how it works and how it fits into the big picture, I want to mention this: millions of years ago life was simple.

Nowadays we live in an extremely complex society that has undergone huge changes. Men live longer and reproduce later – they want to become fathers much later than a generation ago. Their partners are also aiming to become mothers much later in life. First-time Australian mothers for example are now some of the oldest among Western countries, with an average age for having their first child of thirty-two.

Men live in a world flooded with chemicals that affect fertility, from smoking to oestrogen-releasing chemicals that affect the environment and may lower sperm counts. They are exposed to anabolic steroids, alcohol, marijuana (which lowers fertility) and anti-depressants, which affect libido. Depression can be a factor, and there are relatively new sexually transmitted diseases (STDs) that can also affect fertility.

It has recently been reported that sperm counts in men from America, Europe, Australia and New Zealand have dropped by more than 50 per cent in less than forty years. Environmental chemicals and hormones seem to be behind this.

Five fertility factors

Individually men and women can affect their own fertility but let's get started on understanding the road to fertility: what's required to make it work. I have described this in my own terms from many years in the field of reproductive medicine.

There are five *absolute* requirements for fertility.

- **Sperm:** you need to have sperm to father a child. There must be enough (the count), that swim forward well (motility) and have a decent shape (morphology) to do their biological job.
- **Ovulation:** your partner must produce an egg and ovulate approximately once a month. Extra eggs are bonuses, like twins.
- **Sex:** it's obvious, but sex is required for the sperm and eggs to meet. Well, it was for the last few million years at least. Those rules have changed with the advent of in vitro fertilisation and intra-uterine insemination.
- **Tubes:** to be specific, your partner must have open and functioning fallopian tubes. That's where the sperm and eggs meet.
- **Timing:** this is as simple as one, two, three. It helps if sperm (one) arrives before the egg (two), and that usually happens via sex (three). If you are going to have sex for fertility reasons, then having it during ovulation is a requirement.

There are a lot more requirements for fertility, but in my view these are the top five. If there is a problem with any of these factors infertility arrives on the scene, and its arrival is surprisingly common. One in six couples has a fertility problem, and in 30 to 40 per cent of those cases male infertility is the reason that couple is not conceiving. Men are the number one fertility problem in the world but hardly any men realise this. So, let's find out more about sperm and about ovulation.

 ## Sperm

Humans reproduce by sexual reproduction – the mechanism by which two members of a species, one male and one female, produce the next generation. There are other ways to reproduce without sex, but humans do it sexually. Some species just split in half, which sounds painful and is not as much fun as having sex.

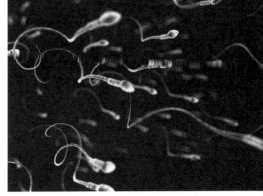

For many millions of years we have successfully managed this, but it has only been very recently that we have managed to understand it.

Eggs have been understood for thousands of years. After all, the chicken came from an egg and everyone knew that the female bird made the egg. But the male contribution to reproduction was not understood for most of civilisation. In the ninth century BCE, Homer believed that women became pregnant through the air or by divine means. Approximately four hundred years later another Greek, Pythagoras, decided that men had something to do with it, but he viewed women as simple carriers in which an embryo developed.

The dark ages descended and for around the next one thousand years the accumulation of knowledge stopped.

Around the sixteenth century the famous British physician, William Harvey, realised semen had something to do with pregnancy, but what?

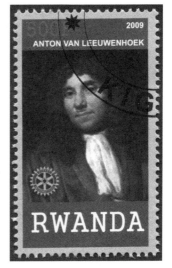

It took the development of the microscope for scientists to begin to understand the role of semen. Antonie Van Leeuwenhoek, a Dutch draper known as the father of the microscope, found that semen contained small tadpoles he called 'animalcules'. Sperm are very small – almost three thousand could fit inside one single female egg.

Things were a little confused back then. Many believed the egg was perforated by the sperm and the egg then provided it with a place to grow. As science was dominated completely by men, this misunderstanding was not surprising. Finally, in 1857 German biologist Oscar Hertwig discovered fertilisation and the idea of a 'blend' had finally arrived. One must remember that the science of genetics was still unknown. A monk called Gregor Mendel was breeding peas around this time and over many years he discovered the rules of hereditary genetics. These ideas were yet to surface in mainstream science.

It has always been surprising to me that back in those times a man and a

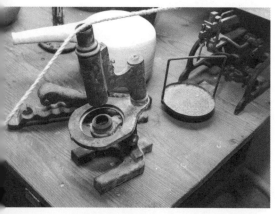

woman could mate and have children that looked like either their mother or father and no one worked out that **both** parents contributed to the child. But then, the Dark Ages were famous (or infamous) for a lack of inquiry or thinking. In the age of enlightenment that followed, mankind got on with some serious questioning of everything.

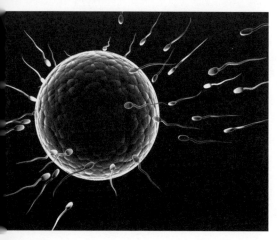

Now we know that the sperm and the egg contribute equally to the embryo. Inside sperm, those tiny creatures that look like tadpoles with a head and a tail, is half the genetic potential required to make another human being. Sperm is a form of taxi that can deliver its vital passenger, the genetic material in the head of the sperm, to a meeting with a female egg. Although nearly three thousand times smaller than the egg, sperm has an amount of DNA equal to that found in the egg.

Sperm, which is made in the testes, is slightly alkaline, which helps neutralise the acid pH of vaginal fluid. Sperm are very acid sensitive, so an alkaline fluid protects the sperm.

The saying 'all you need is one' is commonly heard and while that's literally true for conception – a single sperm is needed per egg – natural fertility needs a lot more. Millions and millions of sperm are needed, and male testicles produce them in abundance. It's also important for the sperm to be in top shape.

 ### A semen analysis

Semen is analysed against three variables. The World Health Organization (WHO) guidelines are the most commonly used, however, they're only guidelines and don't represent the minimum requirement for fertility. Even low sperm counts can sometime be enough for a pregnancy – I've seen it happen.

 ### How many?

Greater than forty million is considered the fertile range, but sperm counts vary enormously and long-term studies have shown great fluctuations. A concentration of fifteen million/ml is the minimum criteria for fertility that the WHO uses.

Be aware that sperm counts, and concentrations vary greatly. If one is abnormal not all is lost. The test should be repeated and the sperm count may well be normal at the next test.

 ### Motility: are they moving?

More than 50 per cent of sperm need to be motile. This can be further broken down into 'rapid progressive' that is, the quick swimmers, down to 'slow' or even 'non motile'. Motility is important and lots of things can affect this; there will be more detail on this later. A sperm not swimming isn't going anywhere.

 ### Morphology: are they the right shape?

More than 50 per cent of sperm shapes are normal. The genetic data is in the 'head' of the tadpole and the tail gets it moving. With a microscope you can also see the small engine-like mid-piece of a sperm, however, the head part is the most important in terms of shape.

The average sperm is rather abnormal when it comes to shape. There are various guidelines for assessing shape and many IVF labs use another criterion – commonly called the 'strict' criterion – where semen is considered normal

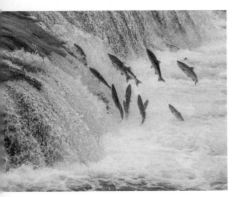

if greater than 4 per cent of sperm have a normal shape. That means up to 96 per cent can be abnormal and yet the semen is still considered to be normal!

A good way to think of sperm is like little salmon swimming upstream. You need enough (the count), they need to be good swimmers (the motility) and they must have a decent shape (the morphology). Fertility also depends on how many of these factors are out of range. One factor out of range can influence fertility. When two or three factors are out of range the overall effect is considerable. If count, motility and shape are all out of range the effect on fertility can be up to eight times worse than if one factor is out of range.

Semen analysis also looks at volumes, pH (acidity) and a lot of other things but for now the big three – count, motility and morphology – are the important factors. For the sperm this is no cruisy late-night drive down empty streets. The journey sperm must make would leave even the world's best rally drivers white-knuckled with terror. Put it this way: in human terms it would be like a man meeting a woman who is twenty-nine metres (95 feet) tall and weighs three thousand times as much as he does.

Just one in a million sperm will make it to the egg. The rest will die.

It only takes one sperm to fertilise the egg, but the odds against them are so high that in a healthy male ejaculation not hundreds, not thousands, but millions of sperm are released.

The saying goes 'it takes just one (sperm) to get pregnant'. And that is true in that one egg is fertilised by one sperm, but you need millions to make that happen.

It's the job of the testes (testes being the plural of testicle) to keep churning

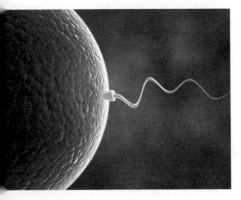

out these sperm throughout most of your adult life. An average male will produce over one to two *trillion* sperm in a lifetime.

DNA, the genetic code that will later join with the DNA in your partner's egg to make the first conceived cell that will become an embryo, later a foetus and finally a baby, is carried in the head of the sperm. Many modern labs can measure the sperm DNA to assess if it is in good condition and not damaged. There are many names for this test, the most common being DNA fragmentation index (DFI). Chapter 4 is entirely about sperm and will help to explain this.

 ## Male puberty

Almost all of us males go through a big change at puberty. What makes this happen? Testosterone does!

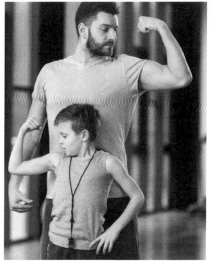

Testosterone is the very male hormone that does amazing things when it becomes part of the equation at puberty. Testosterone is what turns smooth skinned, high voiced boys who want to play with toys into hairy, pimply, shaving, deep-voiced, competitive, strong men who find women (or sometimes other men) very attractive.

Testosterone is made in the testes in abundance. Some helps turn boys into men and some stays locally in the testes to nourish the sperm. In fact, the local testosterone levels in the testes surrounding the sperm are fifty to one hundred times that in the blood stream in the rest of the body. Luckily nature keeps it mostly in their testes, otherwise there might be some serious repercussions – think body builders on anabolic steroids but ten times worse! The Hulk character from DC comics comes to mind.

Testosterone is what makes boys become men. Let's go right back to a male foetus. The male embryo has the genetic blueprint of 46XY. There is a large

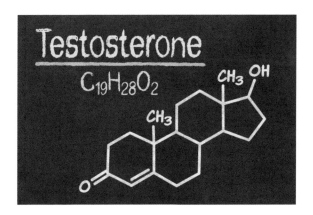

increase in testosterone in the male foetus during pregnancy that comes from the testes. The testosterone masculinises the foetus, developing male organs and changing the brain. After the male child is born the testosterone levels drop down and remain low during childhood.

Boys have reproductive potential but have no mature sperm. So what occurs? Puberty happens, and a genetic switch is thrown in the male brain and the big male engine turns on. A few years later our wee boy is a man. He starts making sperm at an amazing rate of almost one to two hundred million per day.

By now the male has become potentially reproductive, potentially fertile. Mature sperm are being produced in the testes in abundance, and when the whole system is working, strange things start to happen. What are the strange

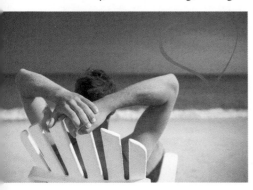

changes in the male at puberty? Girls become interesting. Sexual thoughts enter the male mind, often at an alarming rate. Where once playing, sports and food filled the male mind, a new interest develops – females. Males are programmed to be interested in females. The surging testosterone in the male bloodstream is biologically linked to attraction to the female of the species, and not just any female – the reproductive ones. The wiring in the male brain was all laid down during foetal development. Along comes a surge in testosterone, which provides the electricity to turn the male on.

Strange events begin to occur at night – another basic requirement of male fertility, **erections**, arrive on the scene and waking with these becomes common. The male 'wet dream' starts. Reproductively speaking, all systems are now switched on in the male. Hormones have now reached mature levels and the nervous system has changed. This often leads to some embarrassment but is just another milestone on the path to full maturity. Not surprisingly, wet dreams are one of the least discussed milestones! Adolescent males discuss many things but not that one. Hands up if you ever have?

Strange events occur with the male penis. Whereas once it was a small organ with little use other than to pass urine, it has now grown considerably in proportion to the male body size. It acquires accompanying pubic hair. But what is most interesting is the penis's ability to become erect, to go from a flaccid, floppy state to a hard 15 cm (6 in) structure. And it does this a lot! A state of sexual arousal may occur for up to three hours a day (much of that is when you're asleep).

Masturbation may become part of the young male's life. The cause-and-effect relationship of tactile stimuli to the penis is obvious to the young male; the system works and works often. Biology has linked erection and ejaculation to the pleasure systems in the amygdala area of the male brain, thereby reinforcing the relationship. This creates a biological imperative that encompasses attraction, erection and ejaculation. The purpose of this process is reproduction. Masturbation, like wet dreams, remains a subject only rarely talked about by males. When it comes to reproduction, sex is what men prefer to talk about.

So now we have matured as males. Our hormones have switched on, our testes are producing sperm in abundance, our penis has developed, and erections and ejaculations are part of our lives. Our interest in mature females has developed and our thoughts wander to sex on a regular basis. It's time to turn now to the other sex.

 # Ovulation

Just as male puberty progresses until sperm are made, female puberty progresses until ovulation of a mature egg occurs. This event is signalled by menstruation, commonly called a period – another basic requirement for fertility. Female puberty happens at the same time as, or perhaps a little earlier than, it does for boys. Their surging oestrogen acts on the oestrogen-sensitive tissues and interesting things happen to the female body. Breasts develop and become a great source of interest to pubescent boys. The breasts tell the males that this female is now in the reproductive age group. Males are programmed to respond.

There are many fascinating studies that have considered this area of reproduction. It will come as no surprise that the concept of 'sexy' is merely a reproductive potentiality grade that men give to females. Excellent hormone levels produce excellent anatomical proportions that men can recognise at a glance. If the female's anatomical shape is not the hourglass and is either too thin or more rounded and

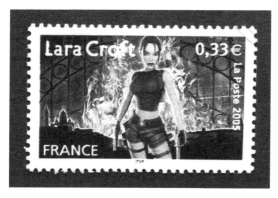

apple shaped, men know intuitively that this reflects poorer reproductive potential. It really is that simple. Modern man has changed some of the rules with cosmetic surgery to enhance breasts, but the basic philosophy still applies.

Chapter 3, on female anatomy, goes into this in depth.

Simply put, sex is a biological mechanism to allow male DNA to fuse with female DNA. This creates embryonic (baby) DNA and soon (in the regulation nine months or so) a human baby arrives. The baby's genetic blueprint was laid down in the DNA it inherited from its mother's egg and father's sperm.

Sperm and eggs must meet. So, we have sperm, in abundance, testosterone, puberty, a mature male and a mature female and sex. Those are some of the basics of fertility.

When things go wrong

Sometimes a road block or detour arrives on the scene and you can get lost on the road to fertility.

Infertility comes down to one of three general possibilities:

CHANGED TRAFFIC CONDITIONS

- **Male factor:** a sperm problem, hormone problems, anatomy problems or psychological problems.
- **Female factor:** a problem related to ovulation, the fallopian tubes, anatomical problems or many other possibilities. Females have a lot more that can go wrong.
- **Unexplained factor:** Sometimes after basic tests we doctors don't know the answer and call it 'unexplained' infertility. There are far more extensive tests to consider if you reach that point.

Infertility is divided into primary and secondary stages.

The definition of **primary infertility** is twelve months of sex without a conception in those never previously pregnant. Remember this number – just twelve months of trying.

NO THROUGH ROAD

Secondary infertility is defined as trying unsuccessfully for six months without a conception in a couple who have previously had any form of pregnancy – a baby, a miscarriage, an ectopic (tubal) pregnancy, even a termination. Not very long is it? Six months!

Every male who must confront his own fertility feels that worry, and is concerned that they might have a problem.

10

| TRAFFIC HAZARD | **Robert's story** |

In my late twenties I began to suffer from anxiety and mild depression. Nothing too severe, but it was making life's issues harder to deal with. I had always kept myself physically healthy, didn't smoke or drink to excess, never used illicit drugs and maintained an active lifestyle. Therefore, I was angry as well as frustrated as to why this situation had crept up on me. While my career was advancing rapidly, I was in a highly stressful work environment that made managing the anxiety even more challenging.

After speaking to several medical professionals, I decided to go on anxiety medication. It wasn't something I was comfortable doing but I knew I didn't really have a choice.

There are challenges with this type of medication. You can't just go off it if you feel you are having a good day, it can drain the energy out of you and, as I quickly discovered, it lowers your libido considerably. When my wife and I made the decision to have a child I still thought it would not be a problem, even if the medication meant that having sex wasn't always on top of my mind. Just thinking about sex took an effort, let alone the need to get an erection and successfully ejaculate for us to have any chance of falling pregnant. However, I realised after more than twelve months of struggling that we were getting nowhere fast. Frustration, anger and guilt were all feelings I was trying to deal with. Why is this happening to us? We have always been healthy: why now?

We went to speak to Dr G, and while my wife got the all clear my results came back with a lower sperm count and low motility – not what you want if you are trying to get pregnant. Dr G was fantastic. He stayed positive, told us to not put additional pressure on ourselves and to change the type of underwear I was wearing (briefs to boxers!).

After several months of healthy living and trying to relax as much as possible my wife told me the fantastic news that we were having a baby.

I discovered that having a baby wasn't as easy as I had always thought.

I am also glad I sought help early enough to ensure I got the right advice and was able to do something about it.

| ROUGH SURFACE | Summary |

Let's summarise the basics for fertility. You need a male and female to start with and for them to go through puberty. Then the top five basic requirements for fertility are:

- Sperm: a normal semen analysis of count, motility and shape is required.
- Ovulation: obviously ovulating an egg is needed.
- Sex: it is still an old-fashioned prerequisite.
- Tubes: open fallopian tubes are a must.
- Timing: having sex before and around ovulation makes sense.

If there is a problem with these basic five factors, then fertility may become infertility. Primary infertility is twelve months of trying to conceive and no previous pregnancies. Secondary infertility is six months of trying and previous pregnancies of any type, that is, a baby, miscarriage, termination, ectopic pregnancy. This medical definition of infertility is unforgiving and comes down to:

- Male factor
- Female factor
- Unexplained

CHAPTER 2

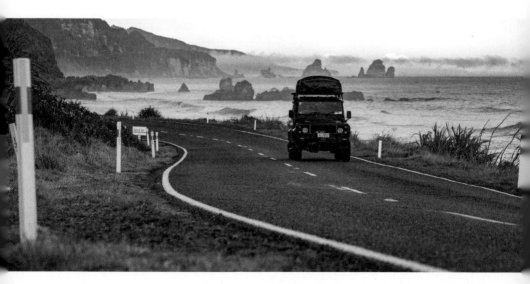

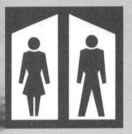

The male body: the reproductive bits

FROM OVULATION TO IMPLANTATION

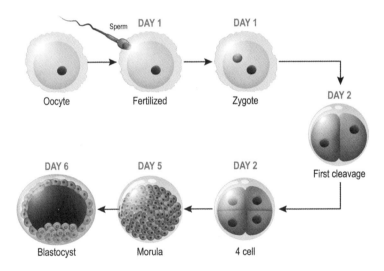

What is it that makes us become men? We know what it feels like to be us, to have male anatomy, male thoughts. But what exactly is the process that produces the men we are? It starts back at that time your parents had sex and one of your father's sperm won the race to fertilise your mother's egg. Your life started, and a series of pre-programmed events got underway.

That microscopic embryo started to grow and on day five it finally arrived in the uterus from the fallopian tube. Once there it implanted itself in the wall of your mother's uterus and settled in for thirty-seven weeks or so. But let's go to the part where you started becoming a male.

In the early human embryo, gonads (the term for either a testicle or an ovary) begin to develop at five weeks.

Idiograms of human chromosomes

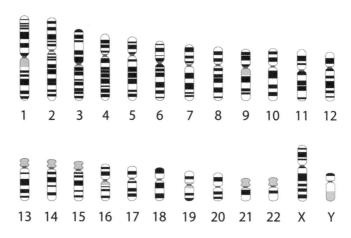

At this stage the gonads are indeterminate – they are not yet sure what they will become. What is needed is a blueprint, and genes are the blueprint or the building plans. The Y chromosome is only found in males, and for males to grow testes to become a male what is required is one single gene found on the Y chromosome, called the testicular determining factor (TDF). It is found in the sex-determining region (SRY) of the Y chromosome. Remember at school when you learnt biology? Girls have XX chromosomes and boys XY. This occurs at six to seven weeks of the pregnancy (or four to five weeks of the embryo). If you don't inherit SRY because you don't have a Y chromosome and you have two X chromosomes, then you become a female and develop ovaries and not testes. It's not quite that simple, but essentially SRY equals development to a male and lack of SRY to a female.

The genes to code for testicular development make up 95 per cent of the Y chromosome. When that one single sperm found its way into the single egg it had either an X chromosome or a Y chromosome. To later become a male foetus, it needed to be a Y-carrying sperm. Anyone who has done it will understand the complicated process of building a house. But a house of bricks is nothing compared to the building of a human.

And just like building a house, mistakes can happen in human development. If there are genetic mistakes there will be problems with making sperm, anything from absolutely no sperm to low numbers.

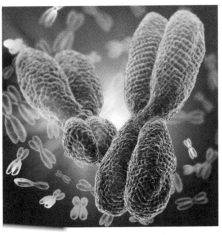

There are genes other than SRY that are needed to develop proper male gonads or testes – some one thousand or so, many of which we don't yet understand.

Early on in males, the **testes** are forming and within them two important components are starting to grow. The first component is the seminiferous tubules (long tubes), which will become the site of sperm production. Approximately 99 per cent of a testicle is dedicated to sperm production. That's what testicles do! They're packed full of sperm-making tissue.

The second component is the Leydig cells, which will produce the male hormone testosterone. These cells will be very busy soon, as production starts to occur around six to eight weeks into the pregnancy.

TRAFFIC HAZARD | Medical terminology

Doctors use a lot of big medical words but, in their defence, the terms were decided upon a long time ago and are mostly in Greek or Latin. To doctors they make a whole lot of sense but to others they are mysterious medical jargon that can be confusing. I'll try not to use too many and will explain them as I go, as they can be quite useful.

For example, the longest named muscle in the body, *levator labii superioris alaeque nasi,* is a favourite. It's a small muscle on the side of the nose. It elevates (*levator*), is on the top (*superioris*) of the lip (*labii*) and is attached to the wing of your nose (*alaeque nasi*). It allows you to raise your lip.

It makes perfect sense to me and is excellent to use for grace at meals.

High testosterone levels aid the **masculinisation** of the male foetus, a process that is quite complicated. Men should never think they are simple creatures. Essentially, the testosterone and another hormone called anti-Müllerian hormone (AMH) work towards making you into a male. A cell called the Sertoli cell, found within the seminiferous tubules, produces AMH, which inhibits any female (Müllerian) development.

The Leydig cells make high testosterone levels that maintain development of so-called Wolffian duct structures (named for Caspar Wolffe, who described the structures in his 1759 doctorate), the epididymis, vas deferens and seminal vesicles. If you want to remain famous discover something first and name it after yourself. How awesome, and it helps if you have a cool name. 'Greening' would add a few difficulties to naming something.

The next section has more information on these. The sperm-making cells (spermatogonia) migrate to the early testes and, by birth, approximately 300,000 spermatogonia are in each of the testes. By the time puberty arrives this number will have swelled to six hundred million per testicle, an impressive number that explains the growth of the immature boy testes to the mature male testes. However, as previously described the huge wastage of sperm during sex means men need these sorts of numbers.

 ## Male anatomy

Men seem to have a scant understanding of their male anatomy. Take for example, the prostate. In my practice I have asked hundreds of men what their prostate does, but I have seldom had an accurate answer except from a medical student or doctor. Hopefully this section will aid your understanding.

Male reproductive system

pubic bone

ductus deferens

penis

spongy urethra

seminal vesicle

bladder

prostate gland

epididymis

testis

scrotum

These are the structures involved in male anatomy:

- testes
- epididymis
- scrotum
- vas deferens
- seminal vesicles
- prostate gland
- penis

 Testes

The testes are the two ball-like structures found just under the penis within a sac called the scrotum. The testes are the male equivalent of the ovary and are packed full of sperm-making tissue. They have an excellent blood supply and are kept at a lower temperature (32°C/89.6°F) than the rest of the body (37°C/98.6°F). Testes move during foetal growth, from inside the body to their exposed and vulnerable position on the outside within the scrotum, by birth, then, as puberty progresses, the testes 'drop' further. Size does matter as smaller testes may indicate less sperm-making tissue. The other tissues in the testes are the Leydig cells, which produce the huge doses of testosterone that sperm require to mature.

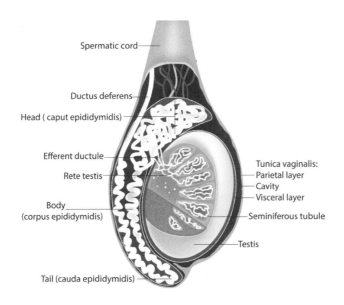

TRAFFIC HAZARD	Testifying

During court trials in Roman times, men were required to swear an oath to the court while grasping their testes that they would tell the truth, hence the word testify. Romans knew a man's testes were important. Even now they are referred to as the 'family jewels' – where the treasure lies.

 Epididymis

Within the scrotum is another structure called the epididymis, a long, single tube some 6 to 7 metres (19-23 feet) long that sits on the testes. When sperm leave the testes they enter the epididymis, spending up to three to twenty-one days travelling along the tube and maturing. There is a small storage area at the end where they wait until ejaculation, which signals the time for the sperm to head down the vas deferens on the journey to the egg. Interestingly, the journey through the epididymis can be shortened by more regular ejaculation.

 Scrotum

The scrotum, the sac in which the testes and epididymis are found, contains blood vessels such as arteries and veins. It is separated into two halves or rooms, with a testicle and epididymis in each. It has a thin muscular coating that can contract, bringing the testes in closer to the groin, or relax and let the testes hang free or further away. The scrotum controls temperature as sperm are optimally produced at 32°C/89.6°F).

 Vas deferens

The vas is a tube that connects the epididymis to the urethra, the latter being a tube from the bladder to the end of the penis that caries urine. The vas is a muscular tube along which the sperm make their final journey during ejaculation, the process of release of the sperm. The sperm pass from the testes up through the groin via the inguinal canal and into the pelvis. They pass over the bladder and join the seminal vesicles forming the ejaculatory ducts that enter the urethra. The operation to cut the vas deferens is called a vasectomy.

 Seminal vesicles

When men ejaculate, the fluid they produce is a mixture of sperm and semen. Approximately one third of the volume of an ejaculation is fluid made in the seminal vesicles, two small tube-like structures just behind the bladder. Seminal vesicle fluid contains the sugar fructose. Men can ejaculate and produce semen from the seminal vesicles but not have sperm; these come from the testes.

 ## The prostate gland

The prostate gland is about the size of a golf ball and is located just behind the bladder. Along with the seminal vesicle fluid, prostatic fluid makes up almost two thirds of the seminal fluid volume and gives semen its milky colour. Also found in prostatic fluid are calcium, zinc, acid phosphatise, albumin and citric acid.

 ## Penis

Last, but by no means least, is the penis. This structure has two important functions, urination and ejaculation. The penis is a hollow tube filled with many muscular tubes that can store blood. When a penis becomes erect blood fills the structure under the control of three muscular layers. The penis becomes erect during sexual arousal and during certain stages of sleep. The urethra travels the length of the penis to an opening called a urethral meatus.

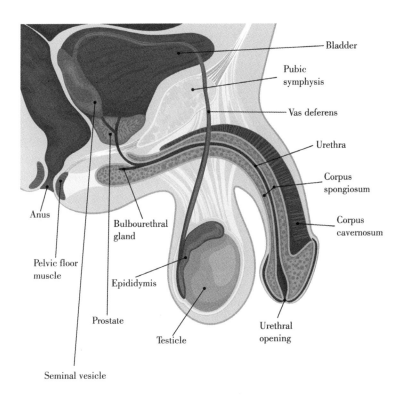

TRAFFIC HAZARD | **How big?**

The erect penis is approximately 15 cm (6 in) long, with a range from 3 to 4 cm (1.2-1.5 in) to over 30 cm (12 in). Napoleon Bonaparte reputedly had a very short penis – if it had been a bit bigger he might not have tried to conquer the Western world. A few famous large penises have been recorded. Gangster John Dillinger inspired the famous quote from Mae West, 'Is that a pistol in your pocket or are you just pleased to see me?' I have examined a lot of men, as one does as a reproductive specialist, and in my whole career I've seen only one large penis that I would classify as unusually large. One. It was 30 cm when erect. 'Bill', to whom it was attached, said, 'And a fat lot of good it ever did me! School was a torment. High school, worse. I never wanted to be a porn star (which is all it seems good for) and there are no thirty-centimetre vaginas, so I can't bloody use it properly!'

Interestingly, in my many consults I have discovered a widely held belief among women that men check out other men's penises while at the male toilet. My (limited) research has found only one country where the men do not stare straight ahead, eyes fixed to not catch sight of one's neighbour's penis. That is Scotland where, as you will know, they have an ancient fascination for large poles.

Most things to do with reproduction and sex start in the brain. I must stress at this point that men's brains are *not* 99 per cent conditioned to think about sex, despite what you hear. Some diagrams suggest this; however, I believe that when men get an idea in their head they devote their full attention to it – call it '**total tasking**', rather than 'multi-tasking'. Sex just happens to be a common idea.

 ## Hormones

A very old structure called the hypothalamus sits towards the back of the brain and releases a special hormone, gonadotropin-releasing hormone (GnRH). This hormone then acts on another gland called the pituitary gland situated further forward in the brain. The pituitary has a lot of functions, making six hormones in all, including growth hormone, thyroid stimulating hormone and others. For reproductive purposes it makes two under the influence of GnRH.

One is a follicle-stimulating hormone (FSH). This happens to be a hormone common to men and women although men don't make a follicle (the small sac in which a female egg grows). In men, the FSH hormone enters the bloodstream and reaches the testes, where it stimulates sperm production by stimulating the spermatogonia.

FSH also binds to the Sertoli cell, found in the seminiferous tubules (along with the spermatogonia), which makes the sperm. Sertoli cells make a special protein called androgen-binding globulin (ABG), which binds the androgen and keeps it locally so it remains in the huge concentrations already noted. Androgen means male hormone and testosterone is the main one.

The other pituitary hormone is luteinising hormone (LH), which has the role of stimulating testosterone production in the testes via the Leydig cells.

HUMAN BRAIN DIAGRAM

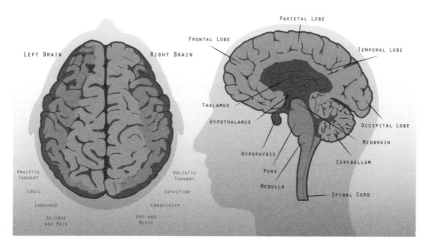

 Sperm production

Hormones stimulate sperm production and from here on the rate of production will remain relatively the same throughout the years until it begins to decline in older age. Men are sperm-making machines, producing between one to two hundred million a day and up to one or two trillion in a lifetime. Each sperm takes approximately seventy days to develop in the testes and then matures during the twelve to twenty-one days required to pass through the epididymis until ejaculation – a lifespan of around ninety days for any single sperm.

Taking three months from creation to release has one major impact: things you do during that time can affect the sperm. For example, a severe fever or a night binge-drinking alcohol may affect the sperm count.

Other factors

There are many other factors involved in making this marvellous anatomy work. Men require a functioning nervous system and a functioning thyroid gland. It's important to grow to a mature size and achieve the correct body weight – being severely underweight or overweight can affect fertility. You need a functioning renal (kidney) system along with all the other biological systems, as well as having emotional balance.

ROUGH SURFACE | **Summary**

The biological requirements for a human male are as follows:

- Y chromosome: that came in your father's sperm and made you male.
- Testes: the Y chromosome made you grow these and they make testosterone.
- Masculinisation: genetics and hormones turn you into a male.
- Male anatomy: you develop a penis, scrotum, testes, prostate and more.
- Other functioning biological systems such as a nervous system and thyroid gland.

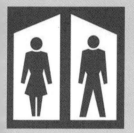

CHAPTER 3

The female body: the reproductive bits

The cliché is that women are a mystery to men and in some ways, including biologically, for most of the last few thousand years that's been true. But we now have a lot more understanding of women's bodies and, given that the only way we can make a baby involves our female partner, some explanation of her reproductive system might help.

Reproductively women are more complex than men. They make an egg, must allow that egg to meet a sperm and be fertilised by it, and then incubate the embryo for nine months in their womb. They grow a 'foreign' tissue in their womb because the baby is half (genetically) someone else's DNA, but their immune system behaves quite differently to allow this.

Women then have a process for delivering the baby (aptly named labour, which most men would gladly miss out on) and finally they aim to breastfeed the baby with the milk they produce.

 ## The X-chromosome

The sex of the embryo is determined by the genetics of the sperm. Fifty per cent of the time the sperm contains an X chromosome and when joined with the female egg's X chromosome an XX (female) embryo results. The other 50 per cent

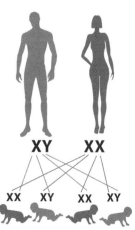

of sperm contain a Y chromosome and thus make an XY (male) embryo. Therefore, sperm determine the sex of the embryo in what is really a random event, genetically speaking.

The development of female reproductive organs begins at approximately six to eight weeks, just as it does for males.

Puberty

Obviously, females need to go through puberty too. The adolescent boys notice it.

Breasts and hips appear: a new height, a whole new shape. Girls take the initial steps towards becoming women in a surprisingly short time.

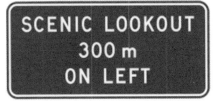

They have a growth spurt (adrenarche) due to growth hormone, grow breasts (thelarche) and start to have periods (menarche) due to the switching on of GnRH, which acts on the pituitary to make follicle-stimulating hormone (FSH) and luteinising hormone (LH). These act on the ovaries to produce oestrogen and progesterone, which results in a follicle containing an egg, ovulation and a period.

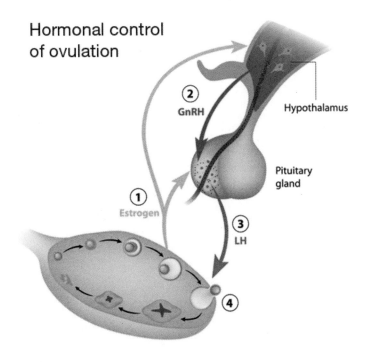

Hormonal control of ovulation

These are the signals of reproductive maturity. The anatomy and hormones are now in place although, socially, girls are far from ready to have babies.

Often puberty occurs in females before it does in males. In fact, the arrival of puberty has been occurring around four years earlier in the last one to two hundred years, which may reflect better health and economic conditions.

Historically, menarche – the first period – meant that a girl had become a woman and many cultures celebrated this event. They were celebrating reproductive potential or, in the great scheme of things, the future.

Ovaries

Ovaries are the female equivalent of testes. Both start life the same way within the early embryo, but the ovary doesn't have to migrate as far as the testes (which must reach the scrotum). The ovaries finish their journey low in the pelvis, approximately at the level of the pubic hair line, one on the left and one on the right. They are small, white and full of early eggs developing. The approximate life cycle of a growing egg is around nine months from early stages through to ovulation. Once a month a small cyst-like structure forms within the ovary called the follicle, about 2 cm (0.7 in) in size, with a microscopic mature egg within.

FEMALE REPRODUCTIVE SYSTEM

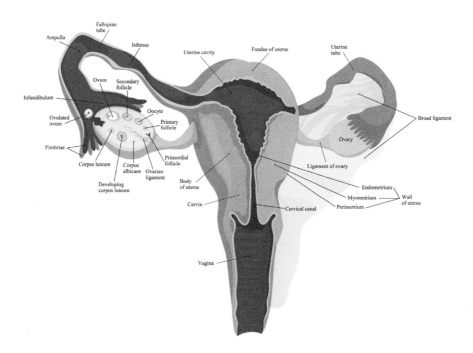

You can see the follicle on an ultrasound scan or at the time of laparoscopic keyhole surgery. The egg is just too small for the human eye to see, at 0.1 mm (0.04 in).

At puberty there are around 700,000 to 800,000 eggs in the ovaries, a big drop from the seven to eight million in the embryonic ovary. During each menstrual cycle of approximately twenty-eight days, around eighty eggs compete to be the one released. That one becomes the dominant egg and it is self-sustaining and suppresses the other eggs – sort of like the front runner in an election can crush the opposition.

Eggs

The female egg is very extraordinary. It is approximately three thousand times larger than a male sperm yet has the same amount of genetic material – twenty-three single chromosomes.

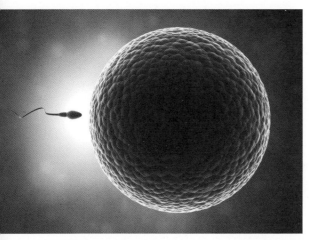

Why is the egg so big, you may ask? Well, for one it contains a whole lot of mitochondria, which give the cell energy. An early embryo needs a lot of mitochondria to get it started and the female egg provides these.

The ovary, deep within the pelvis and enclosed by a strong capsule, has an excellent blood supply. Each month when a woman ovulates (if she is not on a contraceptive like the pill, which suppresses ovulation) she produces a follicle. When she ovulates an egg from within that follicle is released. The follicle remains as a structure called the corpus luteum.

For its short life the corpus luteum has an incredible blood supply, in fact, more blood than the brain gram for gram! If the egg is fertilised and becomes an early embryo, the corpus luteum produces massive doses of progesterone hormones for almost twelve weeks until the placenta is fully functional and takes over.

Uterus

The uterus is a small 6–8 cm (2.3–3.1 in) pear-shaped muscle formed of a body and a cervix. It is a remarkable organ. There are three openings, two for the fallopian tubes and the other for the cervix. It lays midline between the ovaries and is held in place by several ligaments.

The uterus has three layers. There is an outer smooth layer called the serosa to stop anything sticking to it. The thick middle layer of pure muscle is called the myometrium and will one day have a very muscular function – contracting and pushing out a baby. The inner layer, called the endometrium, grows each month, ready to allow the small embryo conceived in the fallopian tubes to implant. If no pregnancy occurs it sheds as a period and the whole process starts again.

If a pregnancy does occur the uterus becomes an amazing incubator. Growing enormously, it provides a safe place for the embryo and later the foetus.

 # Fallopian tubes

Extending 8 to 10 cm (3.1–4 in) from the top of the uterus are two small thin tubes, the fallopian tubes. They are the tunnel that the sperm must race up to meet the egg, the tunnel the egg must get into from the ovary and, finally, the tunnel the fertilised egg, now called an embryo, must move down to reach the safe incubator, the uterus.

Fallopian tubes are divided into different sections. At the end closest to the ovary is a wide opening with a fern-like appearance called the fimbria. It moves close to the ovulating ovary and catches the tiny egg in the ferns. In fact, there is

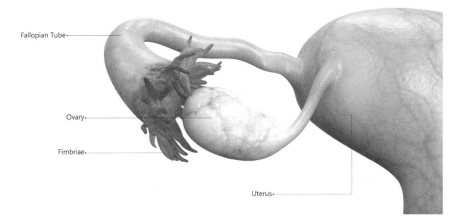

a small finger-like special part of the fimbria that is vital in this process. Eggs don't just randomly and accidentally fall into the tube.

TRAFFIC HAZARD | **Powerful forces**

I have seen a pregnancy where both the left-hand and the right-hand ovaries were missing due to surgical reasons. The tube crossed over diagonally, and a pregnancy occurred! The tube senses the ovulation chemically and moves towards it.

I also once did a tubal ligation reversal but could only microscopically repair one tube. The woman conceived non-identical twins. One egg from each ovary went down the one repaired fallopian tube, met some sperm and conceived two embryos!

 Vagina

A uniquely female opening into the pelvis, the vagina is a specialised part of anatomy. As well as the entrance there is an exit – the cervix at the end of the vagina. It is lined with special tissues that have a healthy blood supply. It is strong enough to cope with intercourse and, especially, the delivery of a baby. There are two special lips on the outside called the labia majora and minora.

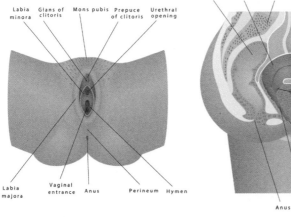

FEMALE EXTERNAL GENITALIA

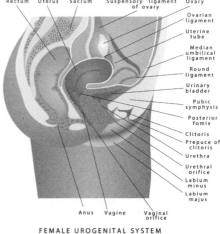

FEMALE UROGENITAL SYSTEM

The vagina is acidic, which helps protect it from infection. It is also hostile to sperm, which must use some tricks to overcome it on their instinctive journey to the egg.

Mid-cycle, around day fourteen, the mucus in the vagina is made up of straight strands all lining up in parallel. A little sperm has a straight run up the vagina, through the cervix and on to the egg. But non-mid cycle, say day twenty-one (of a twenty-eight day cycle) the fibres of mucus are all in random directions. There's no clear straight passage; it's a jungle in there for the poor sperm.

Just at the top of the vaginal opening is the urethral opening from the bladder, and just above this is the clitoris.

 ## Clitoris

The small, almost pea-sized clitoris lies just above the vagina and has a significant nerve supply. It may enlarge during sex, like a male penis, and has a really important role in sex. It may be small, but it is very significant.

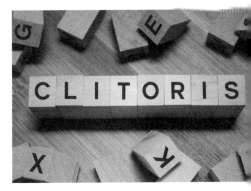

 ## Hormones

A reproductive woman experiences a monthly cycle of hormones, those strange chemicals that do extraordinary things.

Hormones have a profound effect on women in many ways. Mid-cycle, around day fourteen of a twenty-eight day cycle, hormones surge to initiate ovulation and a woman's libido may rise. On day twenty-four or twenty-five she may have severe premenstrual syndrome. When her period finally arrives, she will change again.

It may be a relief to your partner hormonally but also a huge disappointment if she hoped to be pregnant. Remember that human fertility per month is approximately 20 per cent at best. All we men can do is stay positive when a period occurs and be supportive to our partner.

The menstrual cycle

The menstrual cycle is an orderly sequence of events that is divided into two separate halves with ovulation in the middle. The first half, which has the aim of ovulation, is a sophisticated process that allows the production and development of an egg (and sometimes two or three). The second half supports either an early pregnancy or the return to the beginning of a new cycle if pregnancy does not occur.

MENSTRUAL CYCLE

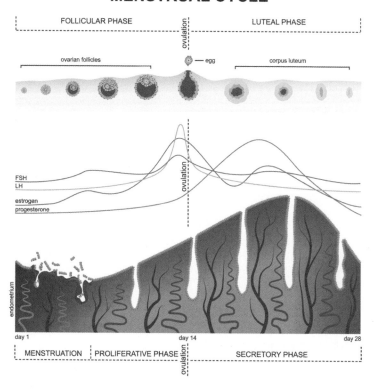

The first day of a period is called **day one** – specifically, the first day of full bleeding, not spotting. Counting from day one is very important in reproduction.

Female menstrual cycles can range from twenty-one to thirty-five days for 99 per cent of women; less than 1 per cent have a cycle length outside this range. Approximately 15 per cent of women have a twenty-eight day cycle. The number twenty-eight is synonymous with cycles purely because of the oral contraceptive pill, which sets a twenty-eight day cycle. Do you know your partner's cycle length? Men should have this information if they are trying for a pregnancy.

Follicular phase

This is the highly organised monthly cycle of producing a follicle, within which is a single egg. During this part of the menstrual cycle a small cyst filled with fluid will develop. Within the cyst, now called a follicle, is a growing egg. Under the influence of follicle-stimulating hormone (FSH) this grows until the follicle is approximately 20 mm (0.8 in) in diameter. The egg inside is just 100 microns in size, or 0.1 mm (0.04 in).

 ## Oestrogen

This hormone is mostly produced in the ovaries and fat cells and a little comes from the adrenal gland. Initially, it is involved with the development of a female foetus, then with puberty and then with the development of secondary sexual characteristics like breasts, fat distribution in the female figure and hair growth such as pubic hair.

Oestrogen regulates the menstrual cycle by controlling the growth of the endometrium. Other effects include increased fat storage, increased uterine growth and increases in bone formation.

 ## Ovulation

A rough rule is that ovulation occurs approximately fourteen days before the next period. Remember that day one of the period is the start of the cycle, therefore a twenty-eight day cycle has ovulation at approximately day fourteen. A twenty-two day cycle can mean ovulation is occurring on day 22 – 14 = 8. That is, on day eight.

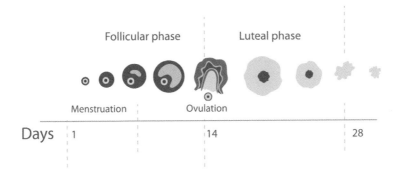

Ovarian cycle

This is not as set in concrete as you might think, and ovulation may occur earlier than expected or even later.

Remember also that the female egg only lives for about twenty-four hours, so sex on the day of ovulation gives the best pregnancy rates compared to sex on other days. Sex the day after ovulation has almost no chance of a conception. Having sex up to five days before ovulation can achieve a pregnancy as sperm can live for up to five days and survive in the fallopian tube comfortably while waiting for the egg to arrive. Timing is very important.

TRAFFIC HAZARD | Seven days of sex

In 2009 at an international conference, ESHRA, in Amsterdam I presented a world-first study of one hundred and eighteen men who had ejaculated for seven days. I presented their semen analysis from day seven compared to their previous standard semen analysis done after three days of abstinence. High sperm DNA damage dropped in most men – sperm counts moderately – while sperm motility improved, as did shape a small amount. It was a novel study and made world headlines as it may have positive implications for men's fertility. *See* the Appendix for more information.

My advice is to calculate the ovulation day then, about four to five days before that, start daily sex and continue for a week.

 ## When is ovulation occurring?

A regular cycle helps but there are other subtle signs. Your partner might have symptoms of ovulation pain called *mittelschmerz*. The rapid growth of the egg-containing follicle causes this pain, but many women do not have it.

The cervical mucus changes from a white, sort of tough mucus to very clear, translucent, stretchy mucus. It is called *spinnbarkeit*, meaning stretchy, making it easier for sperm to travel towards the egg.

When ovulation has occurred there is sometimes a rise in body temperature of approximately half a degree Celsius (32.9°F). The basal body temperature method of tracking ovulation relies on this temperature rise and recording body temperature each morning. Unfortunately, it is not particularly accurate – the temperature rise may occur well after ovulation.

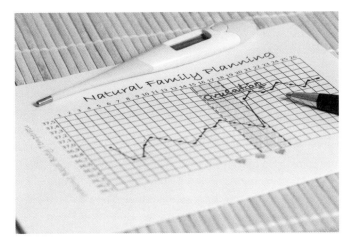

Commercial ovulation kits can also be used to predict and pinpoint ovulation.

TRAFFIC HAZARD | Hidden ovulation

Human females exhibit 'hidden ovulation', that is, they do not show it. When ovulating, female baboons show bright red pudenda, which makes this obvious to male baboons. Other species go 'on heat' and produce hormones called pheromones, which the males smell. The roaring of male bulls for the cows during that time occurs because they can smell the pheromones.

Consequently, human males must have sex regularly with human females to 'catch' this hidden event.

 ### The luteal phase

The luteal phase is the phase after ovulation and before a period occurs. There are approximately thirteen to fifteen days from ovulation to a period, which is consistent. During the luteal phase the hormones follow a consistent pattern.

Seven days after ovulation there should be a rise in the hormone progesterone, confirming that ovulation has happened and is within the normal hormonal parameters. A blood test taken seven days after ovulation will show this. It is important to calculate this correctly, that is, ovulation day plus seven days. For example, day twenty-one for a twenty-eight day cycle, or day twenty-six for a thirty-three day cycle.

The luteal phase involves the endometrium developing perfectly to allow the five-day-old embryo to implant, which is very important. The endometrium must grow synchronically with the embryo; a day-five embryo requires a five-day-old endometrium to implant in.

 ## Periods

A period, or a shedding of the endometrium, occurs once the body perceives that a pregnancy hasn't occurred. Hormone levels return to baseline; the lining called the endometrium is unsupported and is shed and another cycle starts.

Regular periods, occurring approximately every twenty-two to thirty-five days, suggest ovulation is occurring.

To a woman trying to conceive a period is a disaster. She is hoping to conceive and for her periods to end for nine months or more. She will feel her body has let her down and that she has let you down. The best thing you can do is to be positive.

 ## Menopause

Menopause is the cessation of periods. Its occurrence reflects the depletion of eggs until a set number remains. Women who pass through menopause cannot conceive without medical intervention such as using a donor egg. Menopause is not affected by health or economics but is genetically determined. Puberty now occurs at a younger age, but menopause has remained steady at an average of fifty-one years for thousands of years.

ROUGH SURFACE	Summary

- Females need some basic requirements to become female:
- X chromosome: their mother provided one X and their father the other X = 46XX.
- Ovaries: these make the oestrogen and other female hormones.
- Feminisation: genetics and hormones feminise the foetus to become female.
- Anatomy: the anatomical development of female features.

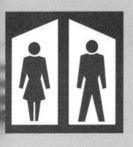

CHAPTER 4

Those all-important sperm

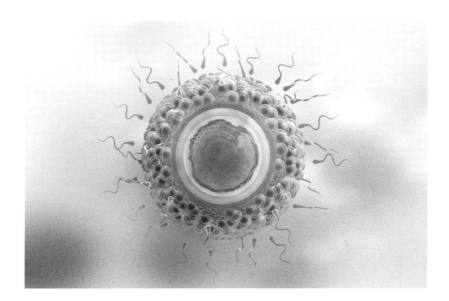

Men make sperm and women make eggs. The female produces an egg and the male fertilises it with his sperm. Let's spend some more time on that uniquely male attribute –sperm. Refer to pages 129-130 in Chapter 11 for detailed information on a semen analysis.

Semen, the fluid that supports sperm, has some very important functions that we will discuss.

Why do men have sperm?

What is special about a sperm? Well, it has two interesting components. First, it has a shape like a tadpole with a head, a mid-piece and a tail. Think of this as the taxi component, a form of transport. Within the head of the sperm is the genetic material, the DNA, which will be passed on. Think of this as the passenger.

It wasn't until 1953 that the **genetic code** was cracked by James Watson and Francis Crick. They discovered the mechanism by which DNA replicates itself, winning themselves a Nobel Prize for their efforts and a place in history.

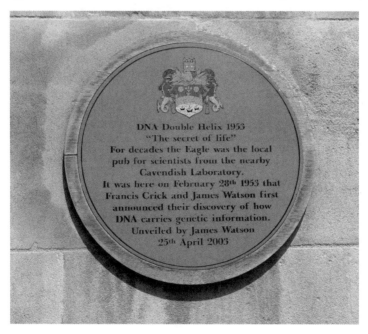

In the last thirty years we have seen huge advances in our understanding of genetics and what is going on in cells such as sperm and eggs. The human genome project has mapped our genetic code and discovered the 31,000 genes that make up a human being.

Human reproduction is about the combination of your DNA and your partner's DNA. A normal human cell has forty-six chromosomes containing the genes. These are twenty-three pairs of chromosomes, with one of each pair originally inherited from your mum and dad. Let's call the number of chromosomes 2n. Half that, n, is in each sperm or egg. Sperm and eggs use a process called meiosis to get the correct amount of genetic material into each egg and sperm.

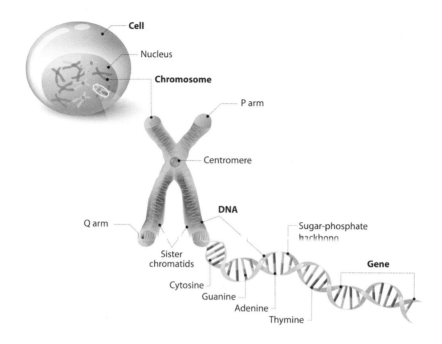

Labels in figure: Cell, Nucleus, Chromosome, P arm, Centromere, DNA, Q arm, Sugar-phosphate backbone, Sister chromatids, Gene, Cytosine, Guanine, Adenine, Thymine

Meiosis is the process of cell division that forms the sperm or eggs with half the number of chromosomes. Meiosis has two functions: it reduces the number of chromosomes and it also recombines some of the chromosomes. Blocks of DNA move about from one chromosome to the other – a kind of shuffling of the deck of genetic cards. This creates genetic diversity and difference in our children. It means that the next generation is a little different from ours, which may have some advantages.

The process of sperm **maturation** starts in the testes and finishes in the epididymis, the storage chamber outside the testes through which the sperm are transported prior to final ejaculation. Human male sperm take approximately three months to mature – approximately seventy days in the testes and between twelve and twenty-one days (but as little as three days) travelling through the epididymis.

Why does this matter to you? Because things you do in your life will affect the sperm and its ability to get your partner pregnant. You might not even be aware of it, but the good news is that once you are you can make choices that increase your chances of making a baby.

Sperm is nature's way of passing on the genetic material to the next generation. Like the tango, it takes two. A male dancer on the floor alone dancing a tango would look a bit silly; certainly I would, and not just because I'm terrible at the tango. When he is joined by a female partner the dance comes alive and something beautiful happens. Sperm on their own look a bit lost but when they get involved with an egg, the dance that makes an embryo and then a child is a beautiful thing to see.

Semen is the term for the ejaculation of sperm plus fluid. A semen analysis looks at the sperm in terms of count, motility and shape. I will cover this thoroughly in Chapter 11.

Semen analysis

Semen analysis can return results ranging from normal through to azoospermia, meaning no sperm. There are many possible variations. WHO recommends two semen tests at least four weeks apart, and the routine test is done following approximately three days of abstinence from ejaculation, to maintain some consistency across samples.

Sperm counts fluctuate greatly, which is normal. The count can be influenced by many factors, including frequency of sex. Fevers can affect sperm counts for months after the fever, a course of antibiotics, some medications and many other things. Personally, if the semen analysis is normal once, I find that acceptable. If abnormal I get a repeat check done four weeks later.

How is semen tested?

First, your doctor will request a semen analysis from an accredited laboratory. A sample is required and there are two ways to achieve it – or three if you consider a biopsy of the testes. Let's start with the simple ways.

A sample can be collected in a special sterile container and returned to the lab either directly (because the sample was collected in a special room the lab provides) or it can be brought from home or some other place. The lab will give instructions on how quickly to get it there.

The second way is to wear a special condom during sex and then take this into the lab once ejaculation has occurred. Normal condoms often contain chemicals that are toxic for sperm, so-called spermicides, to aid in contraception. These might interfere with or affect the semen analysis.

Many men find the whole business of taking a semen sample quite daunting. A strange room, a booked timeslot and pressure cause some anxiety. I suspect the pressure is partially self-induced. What if their sperm count is low? What if they are the cause of the infertility? In some ways it is a test of their manhood. No wonder some worry! I often reassure men to put all those teenage training years of producing 'a sample' to good use!

Semen also may have antibodies as men are allergic to their own sperm. The sperm are perceived to be foreign to the rest of the body, because they are. When sperm are being made there is a recombination of the genes, a shuffling of the genetic pack, to create sperm DNA that is different from the parents' DNA. This recombination of genes amounts to about a 15 per cent reshuffling and is enough for the male's body to then perceive the sperm as foreign or different – it wants to attack it with antibodies.

To counter this effect the sperm grow in the testes and there is a very special barrier between the sperm cells and the rest of the body. The barrier is very tight and doesn't allow cells or toxins to cross. In most men the sperm cells remain safely in the testes or in the reproductive tract during ejaculation; they don't get into the blood stream or outside the safety barrier.

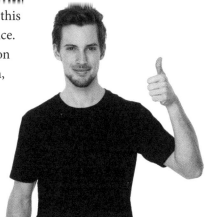

However, sometimes the sperm cross this barrier and an allergic reaction can commence. The antibodies made by this allergic reaction can cross the testes barrier and coat the sperm, causing a lot of motility issues. Men who have had a vasectomy invariably have a degree of this. In cases where there has been trauma to the testes that disrupted the barrier, there may have been an opportunity for sperm to escape and set off the allergic cascade that creates the antibodies.

TRAFFIC HAZARD | Sweaty t-shirts

It might be of interest to mention a fascinating research trial. In the first sweaty t-shirt experiment, Swiss biologist Claus Wedekind set up a test of women's sensitivity to male odours. He assembled forty-nine female and forty-four male volunteers, selected for their variety of major histocompatibility complex (MHC) gene types. MHC genes are used to assess compatibility for transplantation of organs like hearts or kidneys. The more compatible the donor and recipient the better the match.

(Cont.)

He gave the men clean t-shirts to wear for two nights and then return to the scientists. The researchers put each t-shirt in a box equipped with a smelling hole and invited the women volunteers to come in, one at a time, and sniff the boxes. Their task was to sample the odour of seven boxes and describe each odour as to intensity, pleasantness and sexiness.

The results were striking. Overall, the women preferred the scents of t-shirts worn by men whose MHC genes were different from their own; somehow they were less attracted to men whose MHC genes were similar to their own.

Nature plays by some definite rules. Even if we don't know them ourselves, our bodies do.

 ## pH

Semen is alkaline to counteract the female's acidic vagina. The alkalinity comes from the prostatic and seminal vesicle fluid. A low pH i.e. less than 7.0 might mean an obstruction along the vas deferens or absence of the vesicles.

 ## Volume

This depends on many factors but obviously the abstinence period accounts for the variation here. That is why three days is recommended to keep consistency between samples.

 ## Concentration

There is a natural variation in sperm concentration and count. If you multiply the volumes in millilitres by the concentration, you calculate the total sperm count.

 ## Vitality

This is the proportion of live sperm.

 ## Morphology

Human males have few normal-shaped sperm – 2-6 per cent is considered normal.

 ## Antibodies

If there are high levels of anti-sperm antibodies, then fertility is affected by reduced motility.

Trial wash

Here sperm are put to the test in a trial. They must swim up a density gradient of fluid.

 ## Other cells

Sometimes there are other cells apart from the sperm in the semen, such as white blood cells.

Occasionally red blood cells turn up, or even blood.

 ## Other tests

There are a lot of other tests that can be performed on a semen sample because semen is more than just sperm.

 # Sperm DNA tests

Sperm DNA tests are the newest of the sperm tests and are the result of studies on bulls, mice and men by Dr Donald Evenson: an interesting choice of three male species to study! Essentially these tests are designed to study the sperm DNA and discover if there is DNA damage. There are many sperm DNA tests, such as the sperm chromatin structure assay invented by Dr Evenson (*Science*, 240 (1980), pp. 225-38), the tunnel test and the comet test, among others. There is a growing belief that damage to the sperm DNA can affect the fertility potential of sperm and may be linked to miscarriage. The worse the sperm DNA damage, the lower the fertility potential of the sperm and the higher the miscarriage rate in pregnancy.

What could damage the sperm DNA? Radicals could!

 ## Free radicals

The term 'free radicals' describes molecules that can cause damage by attracting electrons; it is also known as oxidative damage. Free radicals are a normal part of the male reproductive tract and are made from defective sperm or white blood cells. Their technical term is reactive oxygen species (ROS). High levels are bad for you.

There are protective chemicals called anti-oxidants in our tissues that can bind free radicals and reduce the damage they do. When that balance is out, sperm DNA can be damaged, affecting fertility.

 ## DNA damage

Why does DNA damage occur? There are many possibilities. First, in some men there is a lack of protamine, the bound protein that is a sort of bodyguard for the DNA. Various genes have been identified as being responsible for this occurring.

Second, after the sperm leaves the testes it has a long journey until it is finally ejaculated. During this journey it is exposed to ROS. There are natural anti-oxidant chemicals to help but sometimes there is damage during the journey.

Smoking and long periods of abstinence increase ROS. By contrast, more frequent ejaculation decreased DNA damage in over 80 per cent of men with high sperm DNA damage levels, in a small pilot study undertaken by me while working in Sydney (a novel theory). Sperm DNA damage can also occur through other means. Infections and smoking can cause a rise in white blood cells and both raise ROS. Scrotal hyperthermia (increased heat) can affect sperm DNA damage by increasing ROS. Varicose veins in the scrotum also have similar effects. Some environmental chemicals such as organophosphates cause sperm DNA damage, as do the volatile chemicals associated with petrochemicals. Cancer can increase sperm DNA damage directly – if you have testicular cancer – or indirectly if you have lymphoma.

The final cause is a bit complicated. It seems that many of our sperm are pre-programmed to die, a process known as apoptosis. If too many of the pre-programmed ones don't die (are rescued from apoptosis) then more ROS are generated, damaging the good sperm.

The sperm's journey

We've looked briefly at this journey above, but here is the full story. Sperm starts in the testes, where it was made. The immature sperm heads out of the testes into the epididymis to begin the slow process of full maturation. It does not know if it is a Y chromosome-carrying sperm (to make a boy) or an X chromosome-carrying sperm (to make a girl). After seventy days of being created in the testes, the sperm have the twelve-to-twenty day journey through the epididymis to mature. At the end of the epididymis the sperm is stored in the distal epididymis.

Suddenly something happens!

Strong contractions occur and pressure is generated – the sperm is on its way to its genetic potential. Rapid movement occurs along the vas deferens towards the prostate gland. The sperm is joined by fluid from the seminal vesicles and the prostate and hurtles past the bladder into the urethra and then violently into the female vagina.

Here it finds itself in hostile territory. It is surrounded by alkaline fluid, but the sperm is safe because of the millions of other sperm and alkaline fluids from the seminal vesicles and prostate. The semen forms a gel almost immediately then prostate-specific antigen enzymes break down the gel. The rapidly swimming tadpole-like sperm enter the cervix via the mucus. If the female is ovulating the mucus is thinner, with parallel strands allowing the tiny sperm to push hard and move forward into the cervical canal.

The first sperm are wiped out by the female's hostile vaginal fluids, but like an invading horde the waves of sperm swim rapidly forward at the equivalent of 40 km/h (25 m/h). They enter the uterus and keep moving, drawn on by subtle anatomical and physiological mechanisms such as contractions. The sperm swim into the fallopian tubes, a less hurdile place. Some arrive quickly, but the first sperm to arrive are like the first wave of soldiers in a frontal assault – they have high casualties. The sperm likely to fertilise an egg come after the first wave. Sperm are being released from the cervix for up to three days after ejaculation. Nearing the end of the tube, they are attracted to a huge egg three thousand times larger than themselves. Signalling between sperm and egg is occurring as the sperm arrive at their destination.

The race is on to see which sperm will be first into the egg to fertilise it.

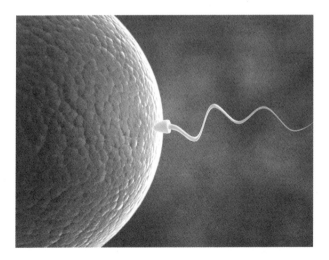

The sperm burrow their heads into the wall and their tails wave rapidly. Suddenly one sperm binds with the shell around the egg called the zona, releases its small container of chemical from the acrosome and enters the egg. Then a reaction occurs that blocks other sperm from entering. Within nine to ten hours

DNA synthesis will have begun; the sperm has run its race and won. Fertilisation begins to occur, with sperm nucleus DNA fusing with egg nucleus DNA.

ROUGH SURFACE	Summary

- Sperm are nature's way of passing on a male's genetics to the next generation.
- Chromosomes in which one is either an X chromosome making a female embryo or a Y chromosome making a male embryo. This is known as meiosis.
- Sperm DNA has recombined to create genetic variety. Sperm carry DNA with a tough task ahead to deliver their VIP load and start a new generation.
- Within semen are other factors like fructose and prostate-specific antigen to help the sperm swim to meet the egg.
- In each sperm is half the genetic code to make a human, twenty-three chromosomes.
- Sperm compete to meet the egg in a wild, dangerous race.

CHAPTER 5

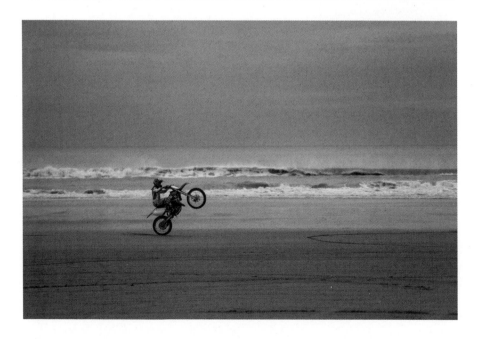

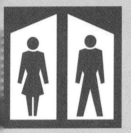

Sex: facts and fun

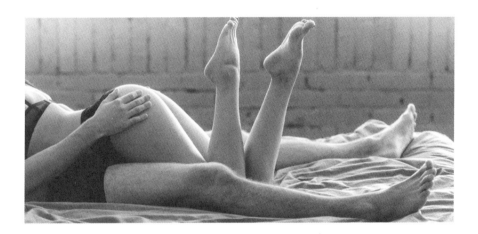

In strictly biological terms the purpose of sex is to get those tiny, yet incredibly genetically valuable sperm into close enough contact with a human female egg to fertilise it and start the amazing process of growing the next generation of humans.

Sex would have to be one of the most interesting topics on the planet, which is why many of you will read this chapter first! It begins with the basics and the biological side of sex. There will be some history followed by some interesting sexual facts.

The second half deals with the *fun of sex*. Noted Australian sex therapist and published author Dr Janet Hall assisted me with this. Sex for couples with fertility issues almost always becomes more difficult. The fun side becomes a chore or even a dread. This part will assist a couple to understand the basics of sex from a therapist's point of view and how to help and improve it, with tips and tricks. Sexual reproduction, where two organisms share half their genetic make-up, is a relatively new method of reproducing. Initially, life developed along asexual- or non-sexual lines. A bacteria or similar cell would split in half and recreate itself with the same genes.

Exactly why sexual reproduction started is a bit controversial, with many theories in existence and not much agreement as to why it came about.

However it came about, sexual reproduction arrived on the scene and it is still here. It has evolutionary advantages that allow new characteristics to develop and undesirable features to be bred out. Biologically speaking, sex finally reaches the consciousness of adolescent males and females at puberty. Before that it has no real meaning and is of little or no interest. That leads to **libido** – the desire to have sex. The desire to have intercourse is pretty much driven by testosterone. Men with low or no testosterone have minimal or no libido, and find erections difficult. It obviously has a significant psychological component as well: young men must learn to control their libido and other urges.

 Our bodies have been hardwired to be interested in sex. Testosterone comes along to provide the electricity.

Libido varies among men. Some have high libidos and some low. Some couples have sex three times a day every day and are very happy, while another couple might be just as happy to have sex once a fortnight or less. Two to three times a week for sex seems the average. Patients tend to underestimate alcohol consumption per week and overstate the amount of sex they have.

Libido can be affected by many factors, but it takes two to tango and couples with differing libidos can have issues. Usually open discussion helps. It is important to see the whole picture in a relationship, not just the small parts. Seeing things from your partner's perspective is a valuable skill, so learn it if you're not born with it. Sometimes it's difficult to come to a true understanding of your partner, as trying to see things from their perspective can be difficult.

 Sex daily for seven days, with ovulation around day five.

TRAFFIC HAZARD	Case study

Many years ago, I saw a lady who was given too much testosterone when she was post-menopausal. She had gone to her GP complaining of a lack of libido that was affecting her marriage, which had always involved very healthy libidos and regular sex. She was given an injection that should have lasted almost twelve months. Inexplicably, she was given another injection four weeks later, which meant her dose was probably ten times higher than the recommended one. I was asked to see her to sort out her hyperandrogenism – having too many male-like hormones.

She had started to grow facial hair, lose scalp hair, get pimples and develop an excellent libido. She became highly competitive at work, had to have the last word in arguments and became quite contentious – quite unlike her previous personality. She started rating the men around her, scoring them out of ten, and watching sport. She loved watching the tackles, the harder the better. She developed a whole lot of male traits that she recognised. 'I really understand men for once,' she told me.

In case you're wondering, I blocked the testosterone with a drug, increased her oestrogen and sorted her problem out over time.

When the hormones are working, and the desire is in place, men and women need some equipment to make reproductive sex happen specifically.

 ## Sexual intercourse

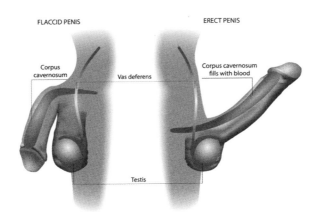

FLACCID PENIS   ERECT PENIS

Corpus cavernosum   Vas deferens   Corpus cavernosum fills with blood

Testis

Sex involves a penis and a vagina, which I have described previously. During sex the penis enlarges due to a complex process. It fills with blood and reaches its full length, which coincidentally is about the same as the length of the vagina. Men require an erection to ejaculate.

The physical act of inserting an erect penis into a vagina is termed sexual intercourse; it is something all animals do. Human mating is considered extremely pleasurable.

There is an amazing number of names for human sex; each couple will have their own terms that they use and find works for them. It's quite an intimate part of a relationship and probably develops over time. I'll leave that with each of you to work on but the term you choose is yours.

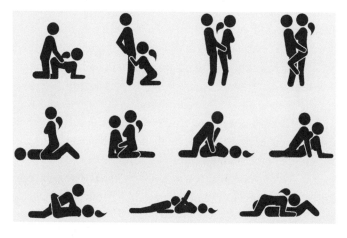

TRAFFIC HAZARD | Historical terms for sex

As this book includes a bit of history, I dug a little deeper into older historical names for sex. Jonathon Green's comprehensive historical dictionary of slang has many:

- play nug a nug (1505)
- night physic (1621)
- culbatising exercise (1653): try that on your partner!
- ride a dragon upon St George (1698); this might have useful regional significance as our local rugby league team in the NRL is called St George
- horizontal refreshment (1863)

Research shows sex in Australia, from entry to ejaculation, lasts on average for two minutes and fifteen seconds. At least human mating is better than what goes on with other animals and insects. Male cats have barbs on their penis to hold the penis in the vagina – hence the screaming of mating cats. The male black widow spider gets devoured by the female after they mate, and yet they still do it!

Sexual intercourse has the role of getting the sperm deep inside the vagina near the opening called the cervix.

There can be a lot of problems with intercourse, ranging from lack of libido, impotence, premature ejaculation, pain during sex (called dyspareunia and often due to a condition called endometriosis), through to vaginal spasms and pain during sex called vaginismus. IVF can be used to help couples conceive when sexual intercourse is not possible.

 # Ejaculation

A male orgasm is a prerequisite for pregnancy in the natural world. In IVF terms it is not quite as important, as a testicular biopsy can retrieve sperm. The process of a male orgasm is a series of rhythmic contractions that produces a forceful ejaculation of seminal fluid combining sperm and fluid from the prostate and seminal vesicles. At the same time as the ejaculation, the prostate blocks the urethra so that semen can enter the distal urethra and not flow back into the bladder (which can happen with some diseases and is called retrograde ejaculation). Nature has associated this with intense pleasure for a male and this makes men addicted to sex, which is very useful for promoting the ongoing survival of the species. The force of the contractions can expel the semen from 1 to 2 metres (3.2-6.5 feet). In the vagina, it pools at the entrance to the cervix in the posterior vagina.

At this point if you're trying to become pregnant it is probably best for your female partner to stay in bed for some time and avoid going to the toilet.

Female ejaculation is quite different. In the 1950s the pioneers of research into sex, Masters and Johnson, studied female orgasm. They filmed an orgasm inside a test subject and saw the cervix dip down into a pool of semen rhythmically as if to suck semen up into the uterus.

 # Sperm DNA damage

When Gary presented to me with a high sperm DNA damage rate, I tried a novel technique: I asked him to ejaculate daily for seven days and we would test his semen on the seventh day. The primary aim was to see what happened to his sperm DNA damage if it transited through the epididymis quicker and had less exposure to free radicals. The secondary aim was to see what happened to his semen parameters: count, motility and morphology (shape).

This simple concept occurred to me when I found that animal studies suggested reduced DNA damage during mating season. Older men with higher abstinence periods showed increased DNA damage. Given we believe about 80 per cent of sperm DNA damage occurs outside the testes, our preliminary study suggested about an 80 per cent improvement with more frequent ejaculation.

In our study, the participants ejaculated once a day for seven days.

We noted an improvement in sperm motility, no real change in shape (not surprising as sperm are made in the testes) and lower sperm counts, which nevertheless stayed in the WHO normal zone. A long-term study of live birth rates is needed to show any clinical effect.

Why seven days, you are asking? The Goldilocks principle: not too much, not too little. Seven days seems manageable for most men and would show us an effect during the research.

Since then we have studied hundreds of men who all followed the same protocol. Ejaculation for seven days reduced the DNA damage in over 80 per cent of the participants. Significantly, sperm counts dropped from two hundred million to eighty million (which is still good) but motility improved. Morphology showed a trend to improving.

A lot more studies are obviously required.

Frequency and timing

How often? The universal advice given couples seems to be generally that every second day for sex is about right, which may have originated from early Jewish texts such as the Talmud and ketubah. Historically there have been many animal studies in veterinary science and animal husbandry that indicate the optimal rates for sex to achieve the best pregnancy rates. Most farmers would probably be aware of the rates, however, for humans there are very few studies.

There is excellent evidence in studies on stallions and many other animals that frequent ejaculation improved pregnancy rates. My advice to couples is to have sex daily for seven days, aiming to have ovulation around day five or six – given that ovulation days vary a bit this means you won't miss it.

A couple just starting out on the road to making a family would almost certainly not find this difficult. However, a couple two years down the long road of infertility might need the blue pill, Viagra, to help.

When is the best time to have sex? The best possible time is on the day of ovulation, as studies have shown the highest pregnancy rates occur after sex on this day. As I have mentioned, the day after ovulation is almost useless but the days before have some hope because the egg lives between twelve and twenty-four hours.

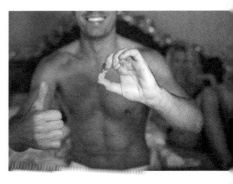

While working in London I met a lovely couple, both professors, who had been trying to conceive for three years. They explained to me in detail how they waited for two days after ovulation to start having sex to be sure the egg was there. Unsurprisingly, their potential pregnancy rate was zero. Their area of expertise was not biology and some simple biological explanation was given to have sex earlier in the female cycle and particularly on ovulation day. They were soon pregnant.

While the egg can only survive for twenty-four hours, the male sperm can last up to five days. I once had a couple who were doing follicular tracking, which is where we use ultrasound and blood tests to track exactly when the female partner is going to ovulate. Her husband was in the armed forces and soon to ship out to combat in Afghanistan. Sadly, her stress and worries meant she didn't ovulate on the normal day of her cycle and he left without ovulation happening in time. She ovulated five days after he left. Surprisingly, her period never arrived – two pink lines denoting a positive pregnancy test appeared on the test stick. It was amazing that their last night of sex, five days before she ovulated, did the trick. There are some excellent animal studies from Professor Sarah Robertson in Adelaide, Australia, showing that seminal fluid is a potent signalling agent that can influence the female reproductive physiology to improve chances of conception and pregnancy success. I tell my patients to take advantage of this physiological effect. What it means in the natural setting is that seminal fluid is useful not just for sperm but to 'prime' the female to improve pregnancy chances.

 Have a few days off, then have sex for a few days between the fourth and seventh day after ovulation.

The fun of sex

It is said that love is a biological trick to get humans to breed. We fall in love with someone to breed with them and pass on our genes; we are programmed to do this. You can bypass the falling-in-love bit and just breed with someone – have sex and get a pregnancy started and a whole new human starts up – but love has other advantages.

You form strong attachments with your partner, stay with them and nurture and support each other. This is also advantageous to children, even after they grow up and leave. You might end up as grandparents. Sex is a part of love; it's not all about breeding. Couples with no children, children who have moved out of home and grandparents all enjoy the sex side of love.

However, until 1978, when we finally worked out how to make babies without sex by using IVF, we have had to have sex to achieve a pregnancy. There has been one famous immaculate conception celebrated every 25 December, and a few other interesting mentions in ancient texts of strange occurrences that produced babies, but for the most part good old sex has been the mechanism for procreation.

This brings me to you, the infertile group. For the last few months or years you have tried this ancient procreation method and have performed the correct methodology of copulation as best you can, but there is no pregnancy. You finally decide to see an infertility specialist. Surprisingly, and rather shockingly, he hands over some condoms and tells you to stop trying to get pregnant and take a holiday from reproduction.

It is often a relief. Phew, you think, thank goodness! I can stop all this never-ending ovulation tracking for a bit, 'the stick's blue dear, get my pants off' and so on. For two or three years, monthly, the demands of turning up, looking interested in sex, getting a manly erection and then finally 'coming' to the party and ejaculating has been your life. Wearing a condom for a month or two (not literally) means that you two can have sex for sex's sake and stop worrying whether this month will be the month you finally fall pregnant. It's a holiday from the chore of sex for procreation. It's sex for fun.

If love is a biological trick to get humans to breed, then sex is a sneaky method to make the mechanical part of love fun for humans.

Sex is a significant part and is supposed to be fun.

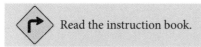 Read the instruction book.

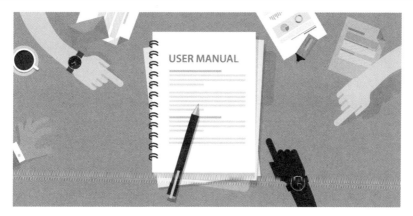

It's easy driving in normal circumstances. But imagine you're put in a Formula 1 car doing 300 km/h (186 m/h) in a race, then it becomes foggy and starts to rain. You need some extra instructions to handle a situation like that and likewise you need extra information to handle the stress that infertility brings to a relationship.

As with many things in life, when the going gets tough you should *read the instruction book*. Sex is like that: if it's not easy and simple any more or never was, get some advice. Read something.

Male and female sexual perspectives

Dr Janet Hall (www.drjanethall.com.au) has written many books and articles about sex and has generously given me permission to quote her work here.

Let's start with Janet's view of a couple's differing perspectives.

Men and sex	Women and sex
Meaning of sex	
Sex = love = ejaculation/orgasm	Sex = love = intimacy
Lust alone is often okay	Only bad girls are lusty
Greatest fears about sex	
Rejection/failure/incompetence	No romance/not being desirable
Timing	
Any time is good/quickies are good	Fussy about time/don't like quickies

Place	
Any place is good	Very cautious about the place
Self-image	
I'm a fine figure of a man	I'm too fat and not pretty
Sexual ego	
Important: to proudly give a woman an orgasm	Insecure: easy for him to orgasm, hard for me
Age of maximum libido	
Fourteen to thirty years	Thirty to fifty years
Speed in sex	
Fast	Slow
Genital focus	
Very high	Like being touched all over first
Attitude to kissing	
Only great when no sex	Always great, means he loves me
Drive to have orgasm in sex	
Very high	Not necessary for fulfilment
Cause of orgasms	
Usually from penile ejaculation	Usually clitoral
Interest in foreplay	
Often boring	Very important
Interest in after play/bonding	
Often boring: he comes, he's finished	Very important: talk to me
Interest in sexual positions	
Curious to try it at least once	Fearful of pain and exposure
Interest in adventurous/risky sex	
Often high	Often low (safety important)
Interest in fantasies	
Often high/useful for masturbation	Often low/sometimes for masturbation
Interest in masturbation	
High, up to 95 per cent still do during a relationship	Probably moderate: 75 per cent of singles do

Interest in pornography	
Often high, used during masturbation	Often low, makes her feel cheap
Interest in sex toys	
Often high	Probably moderate
Best turn-on	
Mostly visual	Mostly auditory
Interest in novelty of technique	
Sticks to routine, doing it right	Likes spontaneity, shows caring
Effect of tiredness/stress	
Sex used as a stress release	Mostly turned off sex
Effect of children	
Not much change	Often drained, not wanting sex

 Talking about sex

Let's have a look at communication between partners regarding sex. You need to have a common language so that you don't make assumptions and don't hurt each other and have a tool that will help resolve difficulties that might arise. Give your partner a written list of your preferred sexual vocabulary.

Remember you come from different backgrounds and opposites attract so you might not share the same words. A few common ones are helpful along with some of your own. For example, 'Bloom County', a comic strip by Berkeley Breathed, refers to sex as 'sweaty snuggles'. It's fun to have your own private, secretive sayings as well as the basic shared ones. The best times to talk about sex are when you're not rushed, can listen clearly and feel close. Never have a deep and meaningful at night; it is not the best time to have those conversations.

I recommend that couples have a quiet dinner out, eat main courses, then have up to forty-five minutes discussing the pre-written agenda, be it sex, illness or any difficult topic (for example, your mother-in-law has just moved in to live with you), then stop, have dessert and go home. It's almost a business lunch approach but it focuses the attention in a neutral place and is associated with a nice meal. When it comes to how to talk about sex, remember there are differences in the way males and females communicate. Prepare your approach in advance and rehearse it in your imagination. I call this *scripting*; having a basic script to follow is incredibly helpful. Here are some guidelines:

- It's important to assess the strength of your relationship in terms of your communication and your quantity and quality of sex.
- Practise requesting sex and rejecting sex strategies – few couples do this.
- Learn to give feedback as direct or indirect feedback. 'That hurts' and 'I don't like it' are far too direct. You might say instead, 'A friend tried this' or 'She didn't like it, but her partner never knew'.
- Try the hot and cold non-verbal feedback strategy. Here you are asked if you like something and asked to give it a hot or cold mark. During sex it's the same. You might say, 'Getting warmer, getting much warmer, getting hot' if that action is working for you. If not use the word colder. If you don't tell your partner, how will he or she know?
- Try the *'appreciate, request* then *affirm'* strategy.
- Try to make some sexual agreements. When you do there must be some guidelines in place: have a non-verbal signal to prevent excessive conflict.
- Have a time-out pause for a hug and verbal assurances.
- Have a physical time out to regain equilibrium.
- Write your thoughts out in a letter.
- Avoid mind reading (men have never been good at this).
- Maintain a sense of perspective and humour.

Record the discussion and evaluate it constructively.

How good is your relationship?

Let's start at the beginning. You were a couple going about your sexual business, not telling anybody. Then infertility turned up. Stop. Let's go back to the beginning. How was sex then and what made it fun?

- Are you soul mates: does being with your partner make you feel like you have 'come home'?

- Are you 'mind mates': do you appreciate and understand your personality differences? Imagine you had to describe your differences to someone else. Writing it down gives it structure and form. If the saying 'opposites attract' is correct, you might see those patterns when you write down your differences. With one couple I once knew, he was messy, and she was tidy, which was no problem until the resentment arrived. Avoiding that required good communication.
- Are you happy with the friendship you have, the trust, the love?
- Are you happy with the amount and quality of romance and the balance of who initiates the romance in your relationship?
- Are you happy with the honesty of your partner, the amount of communication, the equality of communication?
- Is there a power struggle?
- Are you happy with the amount of feelings, thoughts and experiences that are shared and the fun that you have?
- Are you passionately intimate?
- Are you in love from the heart?
- Are you sexually suited: is the chemistry fantastic?

Men are not necessarily good at the deep, meaningful and personal stuff or even knowing themselves well, so for some men, this is confronting and very personal. Terms like 'passionately intimate' are probably rephrased as 'awesome' by men. I can't imagine a man saying to his mates, 'We had passionately intimate sex last night guys.' 'It was great' might be the extent of the comment.

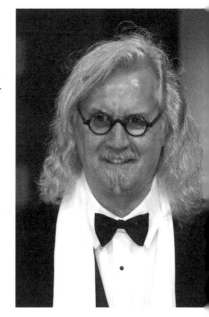

Comedian Billy Connolly, one of my favourite people, did some road trip documentaries and wrote a book about his travels. He reports of the Inuit in North America that they hope for contentment rather than happiness, which is a less common emotion to them. Contentment is preferred to continual happiness because contentment is far more likely, and he thought this was wise counsel. A great 'road trip' would be to follow Billy on his trips around the world. His New Zealand–born wife Pamela Stephenson, who was formerly a comedian, became a clinical psychologist specialising in human sexuality!

Aim for contentment and occasional bursts of happiness, which in fact highlights the happiness and gives it far greater meaning. Living 'happily ever after' is fairytale stuff.

I suggest people in relationships should aim for this, and the same for sexual relationships. If you've been married for five years and have had sex three or four times a week, that's 780 to 1040 times you've had sex. I doubt every event could be called fantastic. Sometimes it might have been a 'quickie', other times two hours of fantastic intimate time together and sex.

Assessing your sex life

With regard to the **quantity** of your sex life:

- How often do you currently have sex?
- Does that suit?
- How often would you like to have sex?
- What days of the week and what time of day?
- In which specific situations do you usually have sex?
- When would you like to have sex?

Some people only have sex on Saturday night, or on birthdays or at Christmas! With regard to the **quality** of your sex life, are you happy with the affectionate touching, the foreplay, the time spent and the quality of the orgasm?

Talk to each other and ask questions such as:

- What's your favourite sexual experience?
- What three wonderful things could I do to you that would turn you on?
- What's the best way for you to orgasm?

Try out the following unfinished sentences:

- Two things I find sexually frustrating are ...
- A fantasy I'd like to act out with you is ...
- Two things I'm afraid might happen if I have sex with you more regularly are ...
- The thing I am most embarrassed to tell you is ...
- One of the worst experiences I've had was ... because ...

Defensive or offensive comments are banned. If you are still tentative about communicating, why not see a good sex therapist to help get the ball rolling?

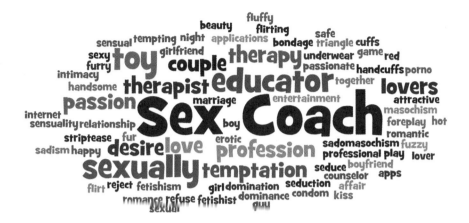

Consulting a sex therapist will provide you both with a place where you can be honest and no points are scored. It should be viewed as the constructive place it's supposed to be. Being entirely open and honest is not easy for some men after a lifetime of keeping stuff buried, and a sex therapist can help with that. Even a single session might be all you need to get a sexual road map.

Sensational sex

How do you have ongoing sensational sex (especially with infertility as a strange bedfellow)? You need to walk the tightrope of spontaneous planning, paradoxical as that sounds.

The secret is to plan to fit sex into your busy lifestyle but then act as if you haven't planned it. Document the plan, then use it as a prompt. Write it down. You may live to regret the evidence you leave behind but at least you'll give yourself the best laugh. Imagine finding the plan years later when you're old, or maybe the kids will find it one day!

Psychologists say it takes thirty days of practice to make a new habit. Remember, we are all creatures of habit, so add something new to your sex life.

A sexy exercise

Make a list of what you usually do and then make changes that force you to do the opposite, such as changing position, to the floor perhaps? Change the instigator. Be creative! However, the best exercise is good old-fashioned …

Kissing

Kissing is the most underrated and taken- for- granted sexual turn on. If you don't think so, remember those early passionate sessions in the back of a car.

Have a decent fifteen minute session and try different kissing styles. The aim

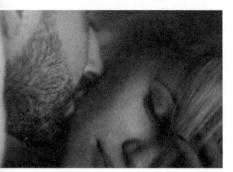

is to give pleasure, not to have intercourse. Vary the giver and receiver.

An infertile couple may become better at sex than a fertile couple, as they put in a decent effort to have wonderful sex. If you become fantastic kissers and practise it a lot, you'll end up fantastic lovers even after the kids finally turn up. Lucky you!

You weren't born a great lover: it takes practice.

 Anticipation

The art of anticipation is incredibly helpful. It starts with realising that women think differently: they absolutely love to think about stuff for ages. They take the anticipated thought out and go over it in many ways and many times. They rearrange the thoughts, look at them from many angles, dwell on them and feel emotionally attached to them.

Men love surprises but females less so. If on a Friday your wife says, 'Guess what dear? We're off on a cruise tonight. I've arranged with your work and you have ten days off, your clothes are all packed, I have packed your favourite three books, your aftershave, your best hat and we are going to have heaps of sex.'

That would be a man's dream come true, but I suspect a woman would have wanted weeks to think about it, plan, pack, tell her friends, daydream about the South Sea Islands more, pick out her cocktail dresses, go to the beautician, dream about the ship's day spa and so on. Surprising her would have meant she missed out on all the anticipation.

 The sweet treats jar game

In this exercise each partner writes anything they want in their love life on a small piece of paper, which can then be rolled up to look like lollies – pink paper for female requests, blue for male. It could be a favourite bit of foreplay, a favourite lovemaking position or a favourite sexual fantasy.

The lolly papers go into the jar and are picked out then read out loud, and you do your best to give that item to your partner. The idea is to give surprises that are exactly matched to your partner's needs. Something that your partner would not like is not allowed; the rules allow for you to replace or remove a lolly if you are not comfortable with the request.

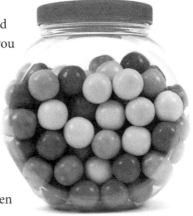

 ## The sexy numbers game

Roll a dice and the highest score starts the game. Each number represents a different erogenous part of the body, so roll the dice again and spend some time on that, say, fifteen minutes. After that you can have full-on sex.

 ## The sex therapist game

In this game, which is for the confident, one person is the sex therapist and the other the client. You toss a coin to see who starts. The one who wins the coin toss calls the 'therapist' (their partner) and asks a question such as 'Can you tell me what my partner's sexual fantasy is?' or 'Could you tell me what the most interesting position for my partner during our lovemaking is?'

 ## More sexy ideas

Here are a few other things you can try:

- a special erotic session once a month, for example, body painting
- a theme month, for example, 'anything but intercourse' (except for ovulation day, obviously)
- experimenting with delaying orgasms as long as possible
- sharing sexual fantasies without acting them out; if you agree, you can then act one out
- creating sex scripts and acting them out

 ## Sex toys

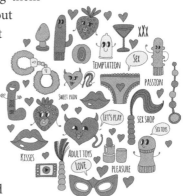

People who play together, stay together. On the next rainy Sunday sneak into the local (or distant, in case friends or colleagues spot you) X-rated shop and explore their range.

The toys don't have to be from a shop: ice cubes, baby oil and so on are easy to get and use. But check out the shop for a bit of fun and agree on trying a few things if you wish.

 Humour

There is nothing like a sense of humour to break down stress. Never ever forget that infertility adds stress: you feel it, your partner feels it and even the dog feels it. Humour will almost always defuse a stressful time. It is without doubt a skill to be learned, developed and nourished.

When you finally get a pregnancy happening and have children you can develop your 'dad' jokes – the terrible jokes that everyone groans about. 'Dad, I'm hungry!' from the back seat of the car. 'Well, I'm Poland. Pleased to meet you.'

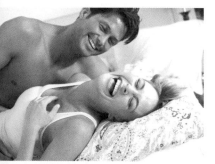

Until you can develop your dad jokes, you need to have some decent jokes. The trick here is to realise that while your mates or work colleagues may laugh their heads off at your wit, partners can be much more difficult to amuse. Remember Jim Carey in *Bruce Almighty*? 'Behind every great man is a woman rolling her eyes.' At least the saying mentions you're great!

You may need to do some homework here and study the topic, but the trick is to script a few funny jokes or sayings to use when the heat's on. I'm going to leave that to you to think about. Work out a few in advance and bring them out (or any spontaneous ones) if you feel stress just before sex, during sex, or if infertility is thumping around the room like an elephant.

 A final word

Sex is designed to allow humans to breed and is also designed to be fun. For the average couple it mostly is. There are some basics to having a healthy, rewarding sex life. You both need to get inside your partner's mind and see sex from their viewpoint. Just start there. Look back at yourself from your partner's eyes and look at your current sex life.

Surprisingly, infertility is often not specifically addressed. Use basic sex therapy advice and add infertility to the discussion. You need to have sexual intercourse around ovulation time. That's obvious, but you can decide on a strategy that works for you as a couple. Maybe you decide to have less sex during the three 'off' weeks and more fun sex around ovulation. Maybe fun sex is during the three weeks when you can't conceive, and ovulation sex is more of a 'quickie'. Do some reading on sex and then discuss strategies that work for both of you.

Remember, infertility is twelve months without conceiving (six months if you have had a pregnancy before). You do not have to wait years to see a reproductive specialist doctor; the longer you leave it the more pressure you will put on your sex life.

Get talking together and add some spark to your sex life. You can try to improve your sex life, which is something that many couples with easy fertility never have to do, but it is an opportunity that will benefit and enrich your sex lives for the rest of your time together.

Like taking advanced driving lessons, developing a sexual skill set will help you along the road to fertility and for the years afterward.

ROUGH SURFACE	Summary

- Sex is nature's way of combining the DNA of you and your partner to make a whole new different human.
- It requires some special anatomy for puberty to occur, hormones to allow sex to function properly and of course two people . . . and mostly it is a lot of fun. Humans are very attracted to sex.
- Around ovulation, have sex daily for seven days.
- Infertility invariably affects a couple's sex life; very few find it fun. You are not alone.
- Read an instruction book about your sex life and how to help it.
- Talk to each other. Work out a plan for better sex that works for you.

CHAPTER 6

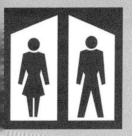 # Factors affecting fertility

The sad news is that many things you do can affect your fertility without you knowing. The great news is that you can do things that have a big impact on improving fertility.

We all know men with terrible lifestyles who have children, but the fact is that lifestyle *can* without question adversely affect fertility. The body builder using steroids at the gym will look awesome, but steroids switch off the testes and his sperm count will likely be zero. The heavy-drinking builder with the physical job might have a sperm count that is okay but his sperm motility is down, decreasing his fertility potential. The well-off couple in their early forties finally turning their gaze to making a family after conquering the business and financial world may have left it too late. The smoker who never quits is doing nothing to improve their fertility situation.

Age

A woman's fertility reduces with age, noticeably once she is past the age of thirty-five and greatly when she passes forty. The female partner's fertility can affect the male partner's fertility. It is fine to say, 'Hey, I have a great sperm count' (and my sperm are just three months old), but if your partner is now forty-four and you've put off trying to have kids for fifteen years to travel or climb the corporate ladder, then a great sperm count isn't really going to help. Keep it in mind.

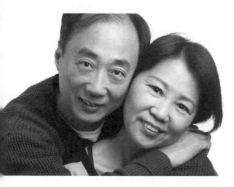

In Australia we have begun moves to try and get some teaching about reproductive health into schools. The female age issue, and its influence on fertility, is huge and a vital fact to plant in the minds of teenagers at school. To a fifteen year old, turning forty must seem centuries away and hard to contemplate but it will happen. Strangely, time moves forward at the same rate for all.

If you are already facing fertility issues you cannot turn back the clock, but if you are already reading this book for general advice it is this: time is fleeting, don't delay.

Refer to Chapter 7 for more information on age.

Obesity

This is more common in the Western world than almost all other factors linked to infertility. A common way of measuring obesity is through body mass index (BMI). The weight in kilograms is divided by the height in metres squared. Say a man is 85 kg and his height is 1.7 m. Dividing 85 kg by 1.7 m² gives a figure of

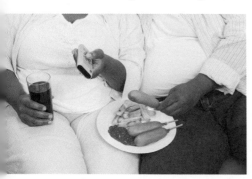

29.4. (In imperial measurements, multiply your weight in pounds by 703. Multiply your height in inches by itself, then divide the first figure by the second figure.) The rough reference range for healthy weight is 18.5 to 24.9, although it is a generalisation. Many weight experts are not comfortable with just measuring BMI as by this definition every New Zealand All Black rugby player is obese. In fact, they just have an awful lot of muscle, which is heavy. But BMI is a useful place to start.

The man in our example is a bit overweight but not obese. If the same man was 100 kg (220 lb) his BMI would be 34.6. When the BMI is greater than 30 the person is obese; if it is over 35 then they are morbidly obese. Morbid relates to illness, and with increasing weight comes increasing morbidity – wear and tear, heart disease, diabetes, hypertension, even cancer. Recent Australian data showed the number one factor causing cancer is obesity, followed by diet and then smoking.

TRAFFIC HAZARD	Body mass index

BMI = weight (kg) / height (m) squared.

The normal range is approximately a BMI of 20 to 25.

For example, a male of 96 kg and 1.6 m tall: BMI = 96 / 1.6 m x 1.6 m = 37.5 (obese).

Healthy weight is 51.2 kg to 64 kg or 112-141 lb (a BMI of 20 to 25).

 How does obesity affect fertility?

Men who are overweight are twice as likely to have difficulty fathering a child as are men of normal weight. They are also three times more likely to have a low sperm count compared to men of normal weight.

There are two mechanisms by which obesity affects male fertility. The first is through a reduction in semen parameters and the second is through erectile dysfunction, where a mixture of hormonal and anatomical factors is at play. Some hormones in fat are metabolised to make more of the female hormone oestrogen, and often obese men are not masculine looking due to this. They have man boobs, little hair and nicer skin, all due to the oestrogen.

Anatomically, testes are designed to operate at 32°C (89.6°F) whereas core body temperature is 37°C (98.6°F). Nature has designed men's scrotums with the testes within to hang free. Large warm fat pads around the scrotum elevate the temperature and contribute to the negative effects on the sperm. A similar effect can occur with tight clothing, such as the lycra shorts worn by cyclists. It is not a hard and fast rule – some men can experience effects on their sperm count while others don't.

 A 7 kg (15.4 lb) weight loss will restore ovulation in 70 per cent of obese females.

Obesity in women primarily affects ovulation. Even small losses of weight can restore ovulation, while a 7 kg (15.4 lb) loss will help 70 per cent of women start ovulating irrespective of the starting weight.

TRAFFIC HAZARD | Luke's story

I arrived at Dr Greening's office after several years of my wife and I failing to fall pregnant. We'd tried everything and done all the tests. Nothing was physically wrong with us, it just wasn't happening. I was a forty-one-year-old man weighing 170 kg (375 lb) with diabetes, high cholesterol and high blood pressure – not your ideal baby-making specimen. My wife was also overweight but there seemed to be no reason for us not to fall pregnant: lots of other overweight people fall pregnant every day, so why not us? Dr Greening told us he could make us pregnant but that he wouldn't now, as I was in a really bad way health wise and it wouldn't be fair to bring a child into this world if I might not be around long enough to see them grow up. Dr Greening gave us a few options on what he thought we should do: it was up to us now. I left his office feeling good about what I had just been told, but my wife left in tears. She'd just been told she was fat, that we both were, but I walked out thinking how good it was that Dr Greening called a spade a spade and told us what we needed to do, so I was on it. Lap-band surgery was the course we both took, with diet shakes and bars for three months to try and lose a bit of excess weight before the doctor would operate. It was not as hard to do as you would think. The day came, the surgery was done successfully and now we would see what was going to happen. After three months we went back to Dr Greening to see if he could help us out now. To our surprise we found out my wife was pregnant. Dr Greening didn't do anything in the end medically to get us pregnant, but he probably did save my life. I was now down to 87 kg (192 lb), my lightest, with no diabetes, normal blood pressure and cholesterol within twelve months. My wife had lost almost 50 kg (110 lb). Seven years down the track we have three beautiful children, two girls and a boy. I now weigh 113 kg (249 lb) but have managed to keep about 50 kg off my starting weight for the last six years and have never felt better. Get off your arse and have a go;– you might just surprise yourself at what you can do. If I can do it, anyone can. Dr Greening, I will never be able to thank you enough for what you did for me and my wife. You gave me a second chance at life and a beautiful family to share it with.

Underweight

Women with a significantly low BMI will almost universally stop ovulating. A small amount of weight gain, around 5 kg (11 lb) and no more, will be very effective. Low BMI in males is rare and has less effect on sperm counts and testosterone.

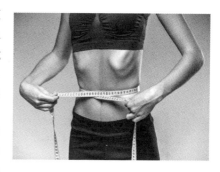

Athletic women have larger proportions of heavier body muscle with lower proportions of lighter body-fat deposits and consequently a higher BMI, which can be misleading. In fertility terms they are often underweight due to this low body fat. Anorexia is a rare but life-threatening condition. A BMI of less than 15 indicates severe effects generally, and always effects on ovulation and semen counts. Fertility is not on the agenda of anorexics.

TRAFFIC HAZARD | Gaining weight easily

My most successful quick weight-gain strategy, which a dietitian patient discovered for me, is to eat your normal diet but in the evening drink a mug of flavoured liquid cream. That's approximately 3,974 kJ (950 calories). In four weeks you will gain 5 kg. Unfortunately, female patients are often more reluctant to gain weight than overweight females are to lose it.

Smoking

The effects of smoking on male fertility have proven to be quite difficult to demonstrate, although multiple studies have shown that smoking affects sperm DNA. There is also evidence that there may be an increase in cancer during the childhood of children whose fathers smoked. The effects may last up to four generations.

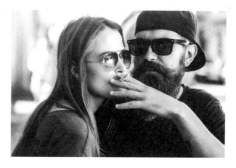

Male smoking can damage not just the semen but also the small blood vessels of the penis. If you combine smoking with other factors that affect fertility, such as obesity or diabetes, it makes for an unhealthy combination.

Female smoking reduces IVF success per cycle by approximately 50 per cent. It is probably also reflected in success per natural cycle, so simply stopping smoking may double the woman's fertility potential.

TRAFFIC HAZARD | A father with a future

A man came to see me with his second wife, who was almost twenty years younger. She was young and healthy but they were having some issues conceiving. He was forty-eight years old, weighed 160 kg (352 lb), was a heavy smoker, a heavy drinker and a millionaire with a successful business. I pointed out that his chances of seeing his kids grow up were slim, and seeing his grandkids highly unlikely. Our conversation obviously struck a nerve with him. He turned his life around, stopped drinking and smoking and lost an enormous amount of weight. He soon became a father. Being a dad and living to see his kids and grandkids was a powerful incentive for him.

Within my own practice, if the couple requiring assistance to conceive are smokers I will often not proceed until they stop. We have a responsibility to do the best we can by our children. Increasing our chances of making them is a start, and taking responsibility for our own health once we have them is another. Quitting smoking is not easy and should not be underestimated; your GP is an excellent resource for assistance with this.

 Save the smoking money!

Another incentive I've developed over the years to help couples quit smoking is very simple: save the money you would have spent on the smokes or alcohol. Do a rough but honest calculation of the amount of money you spend on either or both and work it out as a weekly amount. Open a savings account and deposit the exact amount you've calculated into it each week. Make the account hard to access – no simple EFTPOS card access or chequebook – then watch the money roll in.

The account is for treats, so don't spend it on necessities. Holidays away, a new car, home renovations: all sorts of things can be bought with the money you save. Sometimes it will cover an IVF cycle or more!

 # Drugs

There are many drugs that can have negative effects, such as anabolic steroids. These drugs are used to put on muscle and are generally a synthetic version of testosterone. What men don't realise is that if you take excessive amounts of testosterone, your own turns off. Why should your body make it when you can get it elsewhere in abundance? This switches off sperm production.

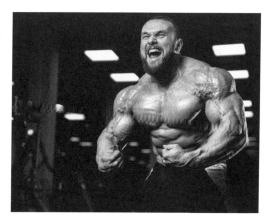

TRAFFIC HAZARD | A cautionary case

A body builder presented with infertility. I used the technique of stating the obvious, as if I already knew, to get him to admit to the use of anabolic steroids in the hope he would assume I had already worked it out and then tell the truth. His sperm count was zero – a huge surprise for him. More surprising and shocking, his liver function tests showed liver failure was imminent. This young man was both infertile and would soon need a liver transplant due to the use of anabolic steroids. As he began to feel worse he took more and more steroids and the spiral into liver failure started.

In most cases, ceasing the ingestion of drugs and allowing the body to repair itself will correct any ongoing issues.

Heroin and codeine-based drugs (now only available in Australia by prescription) inhibit GnRH, so both ovulation and sperm production are affected and testosterone is lowered.

Marijuana is widely used and has a very interesting profile. It has a very long half-life, in that long after it has stopped affecting the brain it is still affecting the rest of the body. When you use it marijuana affects your senses for a few hours only, but the half-life can be up to a week. In men, marijuana affects the sperm. The drug is fat soluble and can cross the testes barrier membrane to get to the sperm. The result is reduced motility.

Ice does have a direct effect on fertility, damaging the tubules sperm are made in. It affects the hearts of foetuses exposed to ice as well. Ecstasy is very similar and has effects on a foetus's heart.

An easy rule to remember: the brain and testes have complex barriers to keep most things out, but if a drug affects your brain it will probably affect your sperm count.

 ## Alcohol

Moderate drinking, that is, one to two drinks per day, does not seem to affect fertility but heavy drinking will. Not only is there an effect on the sperm count, motility and morphology, it also damages the liver, where many male hormones are produced. Heavy drinking reduces testosterone, increases oestrogen levels and

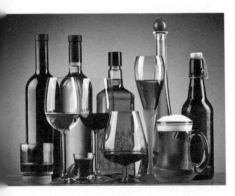 has deleterious effects on libido and erections. Officially, more than two drinks a day increases the risk of infertility by 60 per cent.

Heavy binge drinking can also affect sperm counts and motility for quite some time after the actual event. There is worrying evidence in the Western world of a significant increase in binge drinking, not just the regular drink after work but heavy weekend drinking.

It is difficult to convince men that alcohol can affect their fertility. At the bar or club, they see men who drink as much as they do but have children.

Drug and alcohol effects vary. If you are having fertility issues this may well be a contributing factor.

 ### Women and alcohol

Female alcohol intake is much easier to explain, at least when it comes to pregnancy. The Royal Australian and New Zealand College of Obstetrics and Gynaecology advocates zero alcohol if possible during pregnancy, as no one

knows the true effects of even a small amount on the embryo and foetus. The British Royal College of Obstetricians and Gynaecologists allows up to fourteen units of alcohol per week, that is, two standard drinks per day. The American College of Obstetricians and Gynecologists advises there is no safe amount of alcohol during pregnancy. It would be wise to discuss this with your partner when trying to conceive, as she will carry the pregnancy.

TRAFFIC HAZARD	'We drink together!'

I once asked patients in Ireland about their drinking. 'Not that much,' said the man. 'How much?' I asked. 'Not that much, I just said.' He seemed a bit annoyed.

'Well, give it to me in pints.' (An Irish pint is 550 ml/18.6 oz). 'Maybe forty to fifty pints a week.'

'That's a lot!' I said. 'Not where I come from,' he said.

'What about you?' I asked his wife. She looked at me most annoyed. 'We drink together!'

That is a lot of alcohol for any male or female. It's not good for sperm, for the female or for succeeding with an early pregnancy. A child exposed to those levels of alcohol in pregnancy would be at risk of foetal alcohol syndrome.

 ## Exercise

In general, exercise doesn't affect sperm production, but there are sports that can have an effect. Cycling is one. A significant amount of time spent cycling, with the scrotal temperature raised, may affect sperm production. The bigger issue would be weight: if a woman is a champion runner and slim with a low BMI, high muscle mass and very low fat, she will almost definitely stop ovulating. A small reduction in exercise and a small weight gain will provide a greater chance of becoming pregnant.

 ## Heat

Obesity is the most likely culprit of causing heat-related problems, but other heat-causing situations can occur. Too many hot baths and tight underwear may be deleterious to a healthy sperm count. A few years ago, Professor David de

Kretser at Monash IVF Melbourne invented special trousers to cool the scrotum and improve sperm count.

Abstinence

Abstinence may make the heart grow fonder, but it does little for fertility; there are many research papers that support this. Sperm remaining in the testes for long periods have increased sperm DNA damage and decreased motility. The work environment may contribute to a lack of sex – tired men are not that interested in sex after a hard day at work. Possibly it is driven by the partner's lack of libido due to her busy life. Maybe underlying depression is a factor. Abstinence increases with age, with studies showing that sexual frequency decreases with age. There are multiple reasons for abstinence but ultimately, if the sexual environment results in a long period of abstinence or significantly reduced sexual frequency, this reduces fertility potential.

Obviously if there is a medical condition affecting the male, this will lead to abstinence. When I mention the idea of daily sex for seven days around ovulation to young men they love the idea, while the older guys often look concerned. I regularly hand out a prescription for Viagra to some men to help performance. 'It's not the *Matrix* movie. Take the blue pill, not the red pill.'

Medication

There are a few medications that can affect your sperm count.

Antibiotics can temporarily reduce sperm count. Blood pressure medications can reduce your ability to get an erection. Some anti-depressants can reduce libido (in men and women), for example Prozac. Anti-psychotics for mental

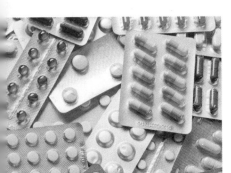

illness and anti-inflammatories can reduce sperm production.

Heavy opiates like heroin and medications with high doses of codeine can create the same result. Men with injuries taking heavy painkillers and anti-inflammatories might therefore have reduced sperm production and low testosterone.

Drugs for colitis and gastritis have been shown to affect sperm also.

There is quite a list, and if you are on regular or intermittent medication it is worth checking with your doctor.

Chemotherapy and radiotherapy

Chemotherapy for cancer treatment has the potential to affect sperm count. There are a lot of different regimes for chemotherapy/radiation therapy.

Radiotherapy has similar effects to chemotherapy. Once again, consultation with your oncologist and fertility specialist is important.

TRAFFIC HAZARD | **Baby after chemo**

I recently managed a case where a young man and his wife were trying to conceive. He surprisingly developed bowel cancer at a young age and required chemotherapy. We discussed this with his oncologist and elected to freeze sperm before the chemotherapy started, as there was a significant risk of rendering him sterile. Sterile means no potential fertility chance. The strong chemotherapy drugs could damage the testes permanently, making sperm production zero.

The patient did well, and twelve months after treatment we used the frozen sperm for IVF with success in the first cycle. There are still embryos frozen from that cycle and some sperm is still frozen. Theoretically, we can freeze embryos and sperm safely for up to 55,000 years before cosmic ray damage to the DNA occurs; a useful fact for a game show. There is a small chance the young man's sperm count will return.

If you face similar circumstances your oncologist and fertility specialist can advise you on what to do with regard to fertility.

Sometimes the rush to treat the cancer is so great that fertility issues are forgotten. Getting a sperm sample can be done reasonably quickly and easily in most cases unless the patient is profoundly sick. Even then a testicular biopsy could find sperm that could be frozen.

It's important that couples consider this in the situation when cancer arrives so disturbingly on the scene. You cannot always rely on the cancer doctors to consider fertility issues as the patient's future fertility is not high on their agenda – saving a life is.

 ## Preconception health

A new field of medicine known as preconception health, which covers the time before conception, arrived on the scene a few years ago. Long-term preconception studies show that men who smoked before their partner conceived may raise the risk of their child developing childhood cancers – probably from sperm DNA damage.

There is also peri-conception medicine, which looks at the effects of actions during pregnancy on the health of the child as it grows. If a mother is overweight during pregnancy she raises her child's risk of having hypertension and heart disease as an adult. If she was not eating enough during pregnancy, this can also affect the child's adult health.

This new field developed from a finding that Dutch women pregnant during a famine in World War II had children with adult-onset hypertension and cardiovascular disease.

As a couple you should aim for the best preconception and pregnancy health possible. Your child will appreciate it!

Environment

Over the years I have seen several men whose fertility was affected by their environment – mostly their work environment. They included men working around boilers at 50°C (122°F), a printer who worked with inks, and a coal miner down a hot mine wearing tight underwear. Other environmental culprits include heavy metals such as lead, cadmium and mercury. DDT has also been blamed, along with other pesticides. One study showed farmers with organic farms who had higher sperm counts. One must be careful interpreting this result; maybe the subjects of the research were in better general health, with less smoking, less obesity and so on.

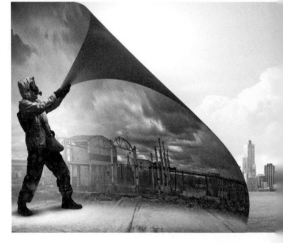

The environmental contribution to infertility is difficult to quantify. Lots of comments are made about it and environmental toxins are often touted as the leading cause in infertility. Natural therapy books mention this often, but cold hard facts are difficult to find. The important fact, though, is that you can control what you eat, drink and put into your body.

Take a universal approach to cleaning up your lifestyle and environment if you're thinking of making a baby. Think about how you can change your environment and lifestyle to best enhance your fertility.

ROUGH SURFACE	Summary

- You and your partner's lifestyle can affect fertility. If you are born with a condition you can't change it, but your lifestyle and environment are within your power to change and you need to change if you are serious about a baby.
- Age is not something you can change but you can take it into consideration.
- Weight: too much or too little can affect both male and female fertility as well as your own wellness throughout your life.
- Drugs: smoking, alcohol, recreational and prescribed drugs may all affect fertility.
- Illness: some things you cannot avoid but illness can be managed to help fertility.
- Environment: heat, heavy metals and other substances may be affecting your fertility.

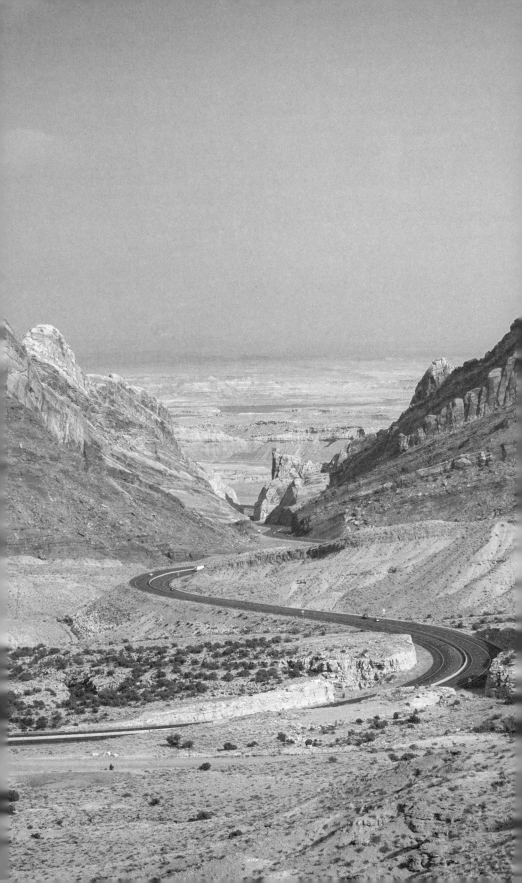

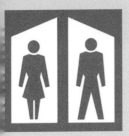

CHAPTER 7

Age

Yᴏᴜ may think this chapter is irrelevant to you because, after all, you can't do anything about your age, right? In fact, with the right knowledge you not only improve your own fertility but also help the health of your partner.

Age is an extremely important factor in fertility, with female age being the most significant factor.

Why?

A woman's ovaries contain a set number of eggs that cannot be replaced, with some women being born with more eggs in their ovaries than others. As the female eggs age they become less fertile. Some women's eggs are of better quality as they age but, inevitably, age is always a determining factor. The using-up of eggs each month during the female's reproductive life depletes the eggs until basically none are left and menopause occurs.

As women and men age they acquire more and more problems that can affect fertility, such as illnesses and injuries. They use medications, they damage themselves by smoking, they have waning libidos and have less sex. They may have busy lifestyles and put fertility aside, but nature waits for no one.

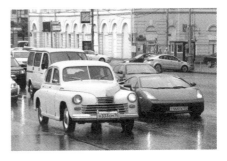

Think about a new car: it has no faults if it has been built correctly, but as time passes and the years go by faults develop. The faults will accumulate as the years go on.

The eggtimer test

The average female during foetal growth will produce between four and seven million eggs in her ovaries. At birth this reduces to around one million and by puberty even more have died. Each menstrual cycle the female uses up a number of these eggs as they compete to become the dominant egg that ovulates. The losing eggs die, and by menopause the female will have practically used them all up.

There is a new test that can measure how many eggs a female has left in her ovary. This test measures anti-Müllerian hormone (AMH), which is made in tiny quantities by each egg. When the total amount is added up you get a figure that can be measured on a blood test and plotted on a graph against that woman's age.

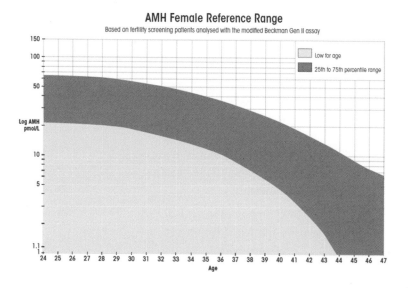

It is a common test and many doctors use it for females during fertility assessments. If it is particularly high that may mean she has polycystic ovaries, and if low we say she has reduced ovarian reserve. It can affect how the doctor thinks about a female's fertility.

AMH measures the quantity of eggs, not the quality. Embryos have been tested during IVF to look at their genetics and AMH levels do not seem to affect genetics. Egg age is the big factor in genetic anomalies in embryos.

A low AMH level, however, might affect the chance of future pregnancies, so it is vital a doctor discusses the AMH levels with a couple once they are known.

Personally, I find it a very useful test as I always think about a couple's family potential, not just this one baby they crave.

 ## The genetics of female aging

A clear example of how female age affects the chance of conceiving comes to us from studies on populations of Hutterites, who were an American ethnoreligious group with no contraception and no family size limitation. Their fertility is very much female age dependent. The number one determinant of success in IVF treatments, which mirrors fertility, is the age of the woman. It is similar for all fertility treatments, but IVF has the best available data.

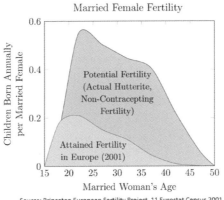

Source: Princeton European Fertility Project, 11 Eurostat Census 2001

Average human fecundity (pregnancy chance per menstrual cycle/ovulation) is at best 20 per cent, which is surprisingly low in the animal kingdom.

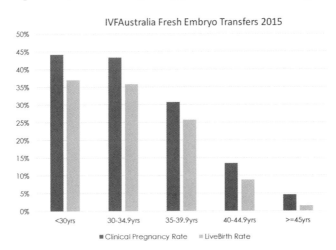

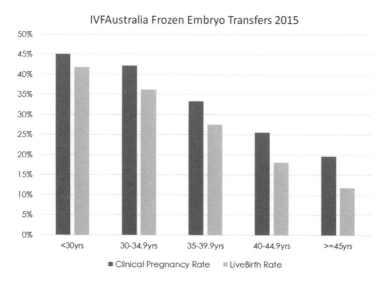

IVFAustralia Frozen Embryo Transfers 2015

■ Clinical Pregnancy Rate   ■ LiveBirth Rate

The older the woman the lower the success rate of pregnancy per cycle started. All IVF units present their pregnancy rates graphically, with the line angling down from age thirty-three and then steeply down from age thirty-eight.

> In fertility terms, female age is a vital fact of which both females and their male partners should be aware.

Telomeres

It starts with a telomere. A what? A telomere! In a cell, any cell, there is a nucleus that contains the chromosomes, twenty-three pairs in most body cells and just twenty-three in each gonad cell, that is, each sperm or each egg.

If you find this information too much feel free to skip ahead, but I think it is fascinating and explains an important process and a point about aging.

When cells divide these chromosomes, which are long strips of tissue, condense, thicken up and begin to align. It is a biological dance with exact steps.

As this happens fine, almost invisible, strings from the ends of the chromosomes align the ends and pull the chromosomes into position. The telomeres are part of this process.

As one ages, telomeres function less well. Mistakes start to occur, and these mistakes begin to have hugely detrimental effects on the chromosome numbers, position and so forth in the cell.

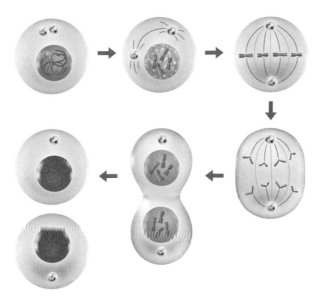

Remember that a forty-five-year-old female has forty-five-year-old eggs and a forty-five-year-old telomere in that egg. When the cell division process starts an egg is chosen to ovulate and is fertilised by a sperm, and phase two of meiosis occurs. The older telomeres make mistakes because of acquired damage.

Mistakes like this lead to either a poor egg with poor fertilisation potential, or a fertilised egg where the division process has gone astray and the numbers or amounts of chromosomes are wrong. That doesn't seem like much, but it has a profound effect on the developing foetus and ultimately on the baby when it is born.

Larger genetic mistakes lead to more dysfunction in the embryo, and they either don't implant, miscarry very early, or miscarry later.

There appear to be fewer mitochondria in older eggs than there are in younger eggs. The mitochondria are the energy-supplying organelles within the egg, the cells' batteries. Some infertility research has tried to improve the mitochondria number by adding more from a younger egg donor. Just the mitochondria are donated in the 'white' of the egg, not the nucleus (the yolk), where the chromosomes are. You might have heard of that as the three-person baby, as it received some headlines.

Chromosomes are numbered from one to twenty-two, and the twenty-third is the sex chromosome. They are named based on a very complicated formula that is based on … size! It's that simple.

This is basic biology to doctors but might be a bit overwhelming to you. You don't need to know how a car works to drive it, even an expensive luxury

Human karyotype

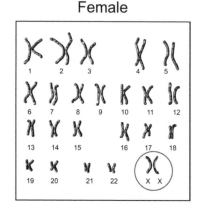

model, but for those of you who do enjoy the mechanics here's more about chromosomes.

If mistakes happen in the larger chromosomes, then there is no possibility of that cell going on to form a normal human. If the mistakes happen in small chromosomes, like chromosome twenty-one, then there is a chance of development but with effects. The extra chromosome twenty-one, called trisomy 21, is the term for Down syndrome. These babies are born with various effects from the extra chromosome twenty-one.

You will notice throughout this book I use statistics a lot and often repeat them. To me statistics are a framework around which you can build a lot of information and on which you can place a lot of value. An opinion is just an opinion, but a reliable statistic is a fact! If you don't know how to interpret statistics, they can be scary.

For example, the statistical rate of Down syndrome babies born to women aged twenty is approximately one in one thousand. For women aged forty-five the rate is one in thirty (that is, twenty-nine women will not conceive an affected baby).

It is important that you understand these statistics. For example, 999 out of 1,000 twenty year olds will not conceive a trisomy 21 baby, however, for forty-five year olds the risk of conceiving a trisomy 21 baby will be one in thirty.

Miscarriage

The miscarriage rate varies with the woman's age, from around one in ten pregnancies started at the age of twenty years to one out of two pregnancies at the age of forty-three.

Miscarriage is difficult, because you have overcome infertility or simply conceived easily and are on the road to parenthood. You have hopes and dreams, then a miscarriage seems like a crash and the end of the journey.

All couples are different. One may be optimistic, one not, one calculating and the other emotional. Some will accept certain odds, and some won't. Some will accept the idea of a donor egg and some will totally reject it. The same goes for the idea of donor sperm if the male has none.

TRAFFIC HAZARD	Statistics and probability

A couple who had had nine miscarriages in a row once came to see me. We found what seemed to be the reason – a genetic defect called a translocation within one of the chromosomes in the male. A small piece of one chromosome was joined permanently onto another.

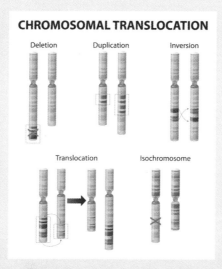

CHROMOSOMAL TRANSLOCATION

Interestingly, the male's grandmother had one live child (his mother) and had suffered twenty-nine miscarriages in the days before they could diagnose the cause or do anything about it.

The miscarriage risk was high. I offered them the option of IVF and pre-implantation genetic diagnosis to test the embryos and replace one without the defect.

(Cont.)

The wife chose to have one more try at a pregnancy naturally before trying IVF. Her words have helped me with many other couples over the years. She said, 'I can go back into that room again, miscarry again. I've been there nine times. I'm familiar with it and I can do it one more time if I have to.'

She didn't have to. The natural pregnancy did not miscarry, and they had a son. The mathematical statistics and probabilities worked out for them that time!

Let's discuss odds a little more. On my desk are a coin and a dice. Toss a coin, and it has a one in two chance of coming up heads. Throw a dice, and it has a one in six chance of coming up a six.

If a couple comes to see me and the woman is less than thirty years old, their chance of an IVF pregnancy is close to 50 per cent. If the woman is forty-one that number is 15 per cent. I show them the coin or the dice. The woman who is less than

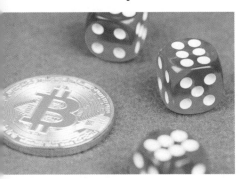

thirty years old has a one in seven chance of miscarrying if she does conceive. At forty-one that miscarriage chance is almost one in two.

You cannot make a dice change its probabilities just as you cannot change the age of a woman. The point is that young woman will need two cycles to get a decent pregnancy rate and fertility treatments like IVF are investing in a probability.

Acquired problems

Aging is something you cannot do anything about, but there are lots of lifestyle choices that can give you a better or worse chance of fertility whatever your age.

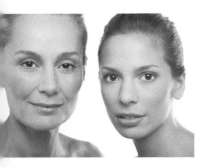

'Acquired' in this case means the defects or effects acquired through ageing, which can greatly affect fertility.

A slim and healthy girl of seventeen with perfect skin is a picture of vitality. She is the same age as her eggs and has not yet acquired many problems.

Skip forward to age forty-two. She may have smoked for nearly thirty years and her photo reflects that. Smoking will have most likely halved her fertility. Her weight has gone up by almost 35 kg (77 lb). At ages twenty-two, twenty-seven and thirty-one she had tubal infections due to chlamydia. When aged twenty-one her appendix almost ruptured and she has adhesions (scarring in her pelvis).

Her periods have become increasingly painful and she may have had endometriosis for quite a while. This has worsened over the years.

Her cervix has had a few problems and her first abnormal Pap smear at age twenty-six meant that by age twenty-nine she had to have a procedure on her cervix to remove abnormal precancerous cells.

She has some joint pains and takes a painkiller regularly, which can affect her ovulation.

From a fertility point of view, she has acquired a lot of problems since she was seventeen. Her age is not negotiable – she is forty-two, and there will be the inevitable effects on her fertility due to damaged telomeres or mitochondrial depletion.

 ## The genetics of male aging

Men make sperm throughout their lives, so the sperm are new all the time. Yet as men age, particularly when they get into their fifties, sixties and seventies and onwards small accumulated genetic mistakes can occur in the cells that make the sperm. Rare syndromes such as Apert syndrome, achondroplasia (dwarfism) and autism occur more with older fathers, and the male sperm is the cause. The increased rates, however, are low.

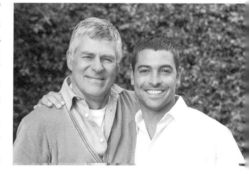

 ### Acquired problems

At the age of eighteen most men think about sex a lot and would love to have sex every day, if not more. It is a biological urge. Suddenly a man is forty-five years old. Sex once or twice a week is enough, and sometimes a few weeks go by before sex happens. He had severe depression in his late thirties and used an anti-depressant, which didn't help his waning libido. His thirty-eight-year-old wife complains about his lack of effort often – she has a much healthier sexual appetite than he does.

His drinking becomes regular. He no longer indulges in the big binges of his twenties but is consistent: a week can see him consume twenty standard drinks between the wine most nights and the weekend beers with the guys. Foolishly, he took up smoking at age twenty-seven and now twenty years later has tried to quit a few times but lacks the willpower. The budget takes a $150 weekly hit from the smoking and drinking but he shrugs it off as he has a good income and a reasonable position in the company.

Shakespeare wrote: 'Alcohol increases the desire but lessens the performance', and it doesn't help the sperm either. Essentially, more alcohol than two standard drinks a day doubles the time it takes to fall pregnant.

The effect of smoking on sperm is less than the fertility effect of smoking for a woman, but male smoking does increase sperm DNA damage. There is evidence it also affects the child's early childhood cancer rates if a pregnancy does occur.

There is little doubt also that as men age their sexual performance declines. As with females, a range of choices and circumstances over the decades will affect a man's fertility.

 ## Medical examinations

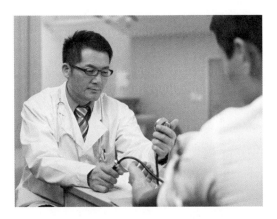

 Females should see a doctor for a medical before trying to conceive. Men should get a medical if trying to conceive from age forty.

I strongly advise all my male and female patients aged forty or over to see their general practitioner for a full medical. If they want to become parents, they need a check-up to make sure they are in good shape. Think of it as a full and thorough car service. You might have undiagnosed high blood pressure or raised cholesterol. You may be on the verge of diabetes. As with the old saying: 'An ounce of prevention is a pound of cure.' Prevention is better than cure and a decent check-up is mandatory. You deserve it and your future kids surely deserve that their parents are in the best possible shape.

Go to the GP and ask for a pre-dad or pre-mum check-up. They will know what you mean.

Before even a standard normal pregnancy all females should have had a medical check-up to make sure vaccinations and Pap smears are up to date, that they are on folate and their lifestyle is optimal.

ROUGH SURFACE	Summary

- Age is a major factor affecting fertility. Even though the female partner's age is number one, men are also affected.
- Age has significant effects on human fertility.
- Anti-Müllerian hormone measures the female's egg numbers and is called the eggtimer test.
- Fertility rates decline with increasing female age, as does IVF success.
- Think about having children before your female partner is thirty-five.
- Put fertility on the agenda by discussing it early in a relationship.
- Look after your body for your own sake, for the sake of your fertility and for your future children's sake.
- Do your best to reduce acquired problems.
- Learn as much as you can about fertility and use that knowledge.
- Get a medical check-up before pregnancy, from age forty for men and at any age for women.

CHAPTER 8

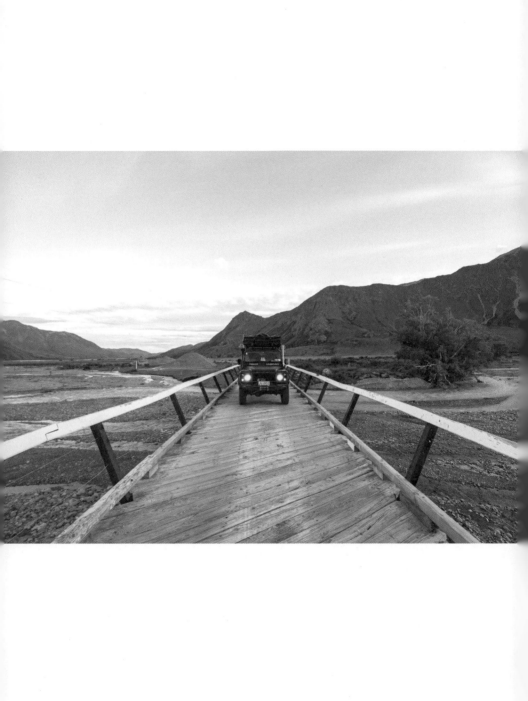

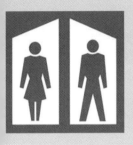

Causes of infertility in men

CHANGED TRAFFIC CONDITIONS

It should be clear by now that men have a significant part to play in fertility problems.

There are myriad websites and textbooks that address the issue of infertility, however it can be quite difficult to find a lot of information specifically about male infertility.

TRAFFIC HAZARD	Infertility on the CCOOAASSTT

Here's a simple mnemonic to remember the causes of infertility in both males and females; there may be more than one. I live on the south coast of New South Wales, Australia and was inspired to come up with this many years ago:

C   Coital: sex

C   Cervix: previous surgery or problems with the cervix

(Cont.)

O	Ovulation: a major problem
O	Other: all the other causes
A	Age: of both female and male
A	Anatomy: you need the right anatomy to conceive
S	Sperm: obviously useful, a must have
S	Sex: repeated twice as it is so important
T	Tubes: the fallopian tube plays a vital role
T	Timing: it is vital to have sex around ovulation

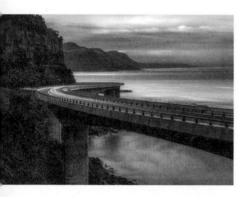

Male fertility problems require men to have sperm and a way of delivering it to the egg. It can be broken down into three issues concerning:

- sperm
- ejaculation
- the vas deferens

When the issue is related to sperm, there are three terms you need to understand:

- normospermic, meaning a 'normal' sperm count
- oligospermic, meaning a 'low' sperm count
- azoospermic, meaning 'no' sperm

You will fit into one of those three categories. If you were born with undescended testes that reduced the number of sperm-making cells, that is a **congenital** cause.

You may have had a huge night out drinking and then provided the semen analysis sample soon after, unaware of the effect the alcohol would have. The result may be a seriously low sperm count and poor motility, but it is temporary – your problem is your lifestyle. In this case, the semen analysis result is **acquired** from your lifestyle; it has not always existed.

Genetic disorders

There are several genetic disorders that can affect sperm production. The Y chromosome carries the genes for sperm production, a vital set of genes.

Infertile men have more chromosomal anomalies than fertile men and not just with the Y chromosome. Men who are normospermic have a less than

1 per cent chance of a chromosomal abnormality. For infertile men the number rises to approximately 7 per cent. The highest risk is in men with no sperm – azoospermia – and can reach 10 to 15 per cent.

Infertile men have up to 7 per cent chromosomal abnormalities compared to men with a normal semen analysis, who have < 1 per cent.
Men with no sperm may have up to 15 per cent chance of a chromosomal abnormality.

Klinefelter syndrome

The most common genetic disorder is Klinefelter syndrome (47, XXY) meaning that each cell has an extra Y chromosome.

The extra Y can have a lot of effects. Men with Klinefelter syndrome are tall and skinny and usually have a wider hand span than a normal man of the same height. The testes may not grow fully, and testosterone production may be lower. The sperm effects range from azoospermia (no sperm) to severe oligospermia (low sperm).

Klinefelter syndrome is the most common chromosomal cause of abnormal sperm count and is responsible for almost two thirds of all chromosomal causes.

Klinefelter is responsible for almost two thirds of all chromosomal disorders that affect the male sperm count, so it is the number one cause by a significant amount. Overall it affects one in six hundred and fifty men, so it is still a relatively uncommon condition.

Some men have what is called **mosaicism**. They have partial Klinefelter with a mixture of 47,XXY and 46,XY. Men with mosaicism may have more chance of having some sperm. Overall, the chance of finding sperm in a Klinefelter syndrome male can reach 50 per cent, according to some studies.

Remember, azoospermia does not mean there are no sperm in the testes. It requires around a million sperm to be made per day (the average is one hundred and fifty million) in the tubules before we see any in the seminal fluid. There may be sperm present, which a testicular biopsy could find.

Azoospermia means no ejaculated sperm. A biopsy might locate some sperm.

The remaining one third of chromosomal disorders is a mixture of abnormalities called translocations and inversions. Simply put, important parts of the Y chromosome are missing, moved or flipped upside-down, making it difficult to read the genetic code and make sperm.

 ## Congenital bilateral absence of the vas deferens (CBAVD)

This genetic disease occurs if the embryo inherits a defective gene associated with cystic fibrosis from *both* the mother and the father. It may cause between 1 and 2 per cent of all male-factor infertility by affecting the vas deferens.

The cystic fibrosis (CF) gene defect predominantly affects mucus production in the lungs. Men with CF almost always have an absence of the vas deferens – the tube connecting the testes with the urethra through which sperm travel. The gene encodes protein involved in the formation of the vas deferens and the seminal vesicles. Some men just have the congenital absence of the vas deferens known as CBAVD. They inherited a major CF gene defect (called a mutation) from one parent and a lesser CF gene defect from the other parent. You need two major gene defects to have full cystic fibrosis.

The good news is that even if a male has CBAVD it is just a blockage (obstruction) problem and he still has sperm that can be used in IVF. Some genetic testing of both partners is required, along with a consultation with a geneticist before moving on to any next step. If the female partner of the male with CBAVD is normal, with no CF gene defects, there is no risk, but if she has one gene mutation the IVF may have to go one step further and pre-implantation genetic diagnosis (PGD) will be offered. That is, IVF units can test each embryo to check if it has two, one or no CF gene defects. Obviously, putting a normal unaffected embryo back into the uterus is the best choice, followed by an embryo with one defect. Those with two defects would not be transferred.

TRAFFIC HAZARD | Cystic fibrosis

The gene for cystic fibrosis is common: approximately one in twenty-five people carry it, so to randomly meet another CF carrier (+/-) gives a random chance of $1/25 \times 1/25 = 1/625$. Then only one of their four offspring will be affected by CF (+/+). Two will be carriers of the gene, like Mum and Dad (+/-), and one won't carry the gene (-/-). So, $1/625 \times .25$ chance of being affected gives a probability of having cystic fibrosis in 1/2500 in the population.

In men with a low sperm count (below five million/ml) a chromosomal test called karyotyping is offered. Because of the risks of passing on chromosomal abnormalities in such men, if sperm are found, IVF with PGD is offered to test the embryos and place back embryos without chromosomal abnormalities.

As each year goes by our medical knowledge to help men with problems like chromosomal abnormalities or others, gets better.

Medicine currently has a lot to offer and it will keep getting better. Never forget that.

 ## Cryptorchids

Most male babies should have both testes in the scrotum at birth, although 3-4 per cent do not. Sometimes one is down and not the other. This is known as undescended testes. Doctors should check this out when the boy is born or is very young. The longer they are left up in the abdomen before having a surgical procedure to bring them down into the scrotum the less chance that the testes will function adequately and produce sperm. The chance of having undescended testes by age one is less than 1 per cent. The aim is to have both testes in the scrotum by age two, depending on your doctor's opinion.

There is also a long-term risk of testicular cancer in those undescended testes and they need to be checked regularly after surgical correction. The risk increases the later in the boy's life the surgery is done to bring the testes down.

The operation is called orchidopexy. Simply put, the testes are surgically brought down from inside the abdomen or inguinal canal and attached to the base of the scrotum by permanent sutures. Failure to bring testes down will almost always result in azoospermia, and sometimes even if the operation is done the sperm count may be low.

 ## Y deletions

The genetic code to build sperm is found on the Y chromosome in an area called the azoospermic factor (AZF) region. If some of this code is missing or deleted the male may have no sperm production or severely reduced sperm numbers. We can do genetic tests on a blood sample to identify this. Men with sperm counts of less than five million are all checked genetically by doing a karyotype.

 ## Sertoli cell-only syndrome

This is the absence of the sperm-making cells. The diagnosis is only made at a biopsy of the testes in men with azoospermia.

Acquired male factor infertility

As mentioned previously, an acquired factor means you were not born with the problem but acquired it during your life. There are numerous causes and numerous ways of dealing with these problems.

An acquired factor may be due to many different reasons:

- drugs, such as alcohol, tobacco, cocaine, heroin, opiates, anabolic steroids
- medications such as chemotherapy, some antibiotics, cimetidine
- diseases, such as diabetes
- trauma, such as motor vehicle accident, quadriplegia, sport injuries
- environment, such as heat in a boiler or cycling
- anatomical, such as hernias, varicoceles, weight gain

 ## Drugs

Over-indulgence in alcohol is a common acquired cause of male factor infertility. Men binge drink more than do women, and for some men this can affect their sperm count. The use of marijuana, cocaine, methamphetamine (ice), ecstasy and heroin can also contribute to male factor infertility, which can be improved with lifestyle modification. It is important to remember that individual humans can be affected in different ways by drugs or medications or even diseases. Your friends may binge drink with you regularly and have no fertility problems, while you do.

 ## Impotence

One of the causes for infertility may in fact be ejaculatory dysfunction. Impotence is the inability to get and maintain an erection. In the context of male factor infertility this would include the inability to perform penetrative and ejaculatory intercourse.

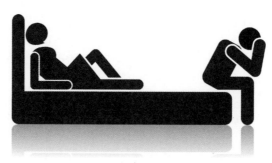

Some impotence is temporary and of no consequence; alcohol or simple stress can affect performance. Up to 50 per cent of men who are forty to seventy years of age experience some intermittent erection dysfunction.

TRAFFIC HAZARD	A simple test

If you have erections in your sleep then your impotence is psychological. If there are none then it is physiological.

Ask your partner to check up on you during the night.

Long-term impotence has two potential causes: psychological or physiological. For a multitude of reasons the man may have a psychological inability to get an erection: work stress, performance issues or even a past history of sexual abuse may be behind it. There is a very simple method for working out if the problem is psychological.

For some obscure reason men get erections in their sleep during rapid eye movement (REM) sleep, the deep sleep where dreams occur. If the female partner checks during the night and there is a full erection during REM sleep this means the male's impotence is psychological. A sex therapist can work out the issues, usually quite easily.

Physiological impotence means it is a functional problem, and there will be no erections in sleep for these men. There are several causes:

- Endocrine diseases: diabetes is the most common here due to the small nerve damage. Hypogonadism (testicular failure) with low testosterone may be a factor.
- Neurological conditions: Alzheimer's, multiple sclerosis, prostate surgery after effects, strokes, epilepsy and para/quadriplegia.
- Medication: there is a long list of medications that can cause erectile dysfunction, from beta blockers for blood pressure to diuretics. Do a Google search on your medications, or better still check with your family doctor.
- Cardiac disease: this is more common in older men with atherosclerosis (hardening of the arteries) due to high cholesterol. A GP check-up is needed.
- Social drugs like alcohol, cocaine and amphetamines may cause erectile dysfunction.
- Urological problems, for example, pelvic trauma.

These causes are quite common, and more so in men with infertility. Over the years I have noted that the longer the period of infertility for the couple, the greater the chance there is a male factor performance issue, ranging from a lack of libido to impotence. After two years of trying for a baby I estimate that over 90 per cent of men will struggle to perform sexually and impotence is common. Without doubt this is psychological, as the continued failure to conceive plays with the male psyche.

I give these couples some condoms to use, as the condoms give permission to take a holiday from the fertility merry-go-round on which they are stuck. Condoms mean zero chance of conceiving, but after two years or so the couple's chance of conceiving is close to zero anyway. Giving them a break and having sex that is not for reproductive purposes is like a holiday from the stress of infertility. They can then return to treatment.

Listed below are some of the more complex causes of male factor infertility.

 ## Testicular failure and trauma

Primary testicular failure is a type of male hypogonadism that originates from the testes. Hypo means 'low' or 'under' as in hypodermic needle, under the skin. Gonadism refers to the functionality of the gonads, the testes.

There are three distinct groups of men with hypogonadism:

- Primary testicular failure: essentially the testes have failed for a multitude of reasons. Consequently, the hormones from the pituitary that stimulate the testes to work are quite high, and the hormones that the testes should be making are quite low.
- Gonadotropin deficiency: in these men the pituitary is producing less or a deficiency of, hormones.
- Testosterone deficiency in older men, because of age.

These conditions may manifest in different ways depending on the cause. Many of the problems will not become apparent until puberty, when the male hormones should be activated in massively increased amounts.

If the testes are severely injured hypogonadism can result. Almost every male can recall an incident of **testicular trauma**, mostly involving sport. I've only seen one severe trauma, which resulted from taekwondo. The affected man spent two weeks in hospital.

 ## Mumps

Occasionally the mumps virus goes to the testes, and if this happens after puberty it can damage the sperm-making cells and the testosterone-producing cells permanently.

If you had mumps you will remember – it causes orchitis, or inflammation of the testes, and the pain is terrible. The chance of azoospermia is rare but oligospermia occurs in around 50 per cent of men who had mumps.

Vaccination of young males reduces this risk. The mumps vaccination is generally given along with the measles and rubella vaccine known as MMR.

A 1998 study by Andrew Wakefield (published in the *Lancet* journal then discredited and retracted) linking MMR to autism was found to be completely fraudulent but unfortunately some parents have still not got the message. This damaging hoax was described by Wikipedia as '**perhaps the most damaging medical hoax of the last 100 years**'. For the sake of your children you need to let go of any doubts you have about vaccinations.

 ## Haemochromatosis

This is an iron storage disease, a genetic condition that means the body stores too much iron, which can affect the testes or sometimes the pituitary gland. Essentially, the gonads reduce or stop production of sperm. Fortunately, it is rare.

 ## Cancer treatments

Chemotherapy or radiotherapy may permanently affect sperm and testosterone production. Storing sperm away before starting treatment is a smart move, and the oncologist should mention it. If not, you should. It can work only if the male has reached adolescence and is making sperm. In fact, anyone can ask about sperm storage as the male with the cancer may be too unwell to even think about it and storage might be overlooked.

I recently helped a severe leukaemic male get sperm prior to urgent chemotherapy by using high-dose Viagra. He deserved a medal for his achievement in the most terrible circumstances and will hopefully be rewarded later with a child.

ROUGH SURFACE	Summary

- There are many causes of male infertility. Some you are born with or you acquired the problem during life and cannot change it. Others you can change.

(Cont.)

- Genetic causes may be diagnosed: you may need a biopsy; you might need a sex therapist. Some conditions may be acquired due to disease or lifestyle.
- Your body is a brilliantly designed, complex biological unit, as is your fertility component.
- The first step in diagnosing male factor infertility is to get the diagnosis, which means a semen analysis. Start there. If there is a problem, you need it to be diagnosed and then try to fix it. The first step is to diagnose the problem.

CHAPTER 9

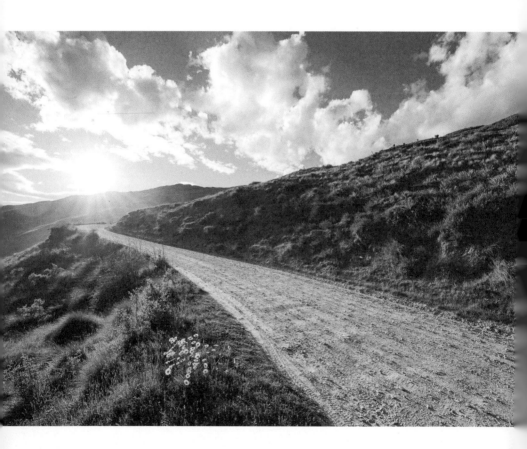

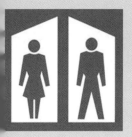

Causes of infertility in women

I rely on my car to get me where I want to go. My car is a technological marvel and I have absolutely no idea about much of it, but I know the basics. Your partner is an anatomical and physiological marvel and you need to know about her.

You may note that sometimes I use 'female' and sometimes 'woman' throughout the book. I use woman to mean a mature female in the reproductive age group. A female covers all age groups.

Anatomy

These are the basic anatomical components:

- Genes: for everything to work a woman's blueprint, her genetic code, must be correct. Genetic mistakes can lead to production mistakes.
- A brain: within this are the hypothalamus and pituitary gland, which make the hormones required to start the female reproductive cycle.
- Ovaries: the female equivalent of testes, which lie hidden deep inside the pelvis. A lot of problems can occur with the ovaries.
- Fallopian tubes: if the egg can't travel down the tubes to meet the sperm a baby can't be made.
- Uterus: a woman needs a uterus to have a menstrual cycle. Once she is pregnant the uterus is an amazing incubator.

Even when all these components are working properly there are other things that might contribute to infertility:

- Diseases: there is a big list but anorexia, diabetes, a ruptured appendix and chlamydia (a sexually transmitted infection) are a few that can cause problems.
- Age: ultimately, age is the single biggest reason for fertility ending. Fertility is high in the young and always drops with age.
- Acquired problems: things happen during life and women acquire problems because of lifestyle choices or through using medications that affect fertility, just as do men.

 ## The brain

For puberty to start the anatomical parts must be in place and they must switch on. Sometimes they don't, and no puberty occurs.

A classic example is a syndrome called Turner syndrome. Only one female X chromosome is present within the female genes, not two. Girls with Turner syndrome don't have ovaries, or if they do they are called streak ovaries and don't work. In this case puberty doesn't happen, because if the ovaries can't turn on they can't make the female hormones oestrogen and progesterone. There are no eggs in streak ovaries. Turner syndrome girls can be given an appropriate hormone to bring on puberty. In the future an egg donor can assist fertility because there is a uterus.

Another example is Kallmann syndrome, in which females don't make follicle-stimulating hormone and luteinising hormone in their brains due to the absence of the gonadotrophin-releasing hormone, which normally stimulates their production, and thus don't go through puberty. It's rare, and weirdly females with Kallmann syndrome lack the sense of smell.

 ## Ovaries

There are a lot of ovarian problems but the one that everyone has heard about is polycystic ovarian syndrome (PCOS). PCOS is not primarily an ovary problem, although the response to the problem is seen in the ovaries. In this case women stop ovulating and instead make a lot of cysts.

Polycystic ovarian syndrome

PCOS is specifically defined according to what are known as the Rotterdam criteria (see the box below). Any two of the three criteria are needed to identify PCOS.

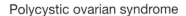
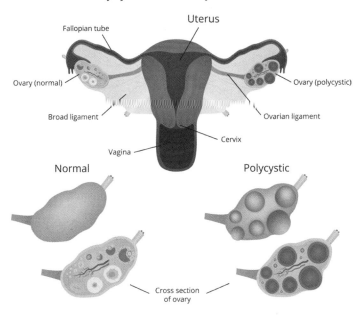

| TRAFFIC HAZARD | The Rotterdam criteria |

- The presence of polycystic ovaries on an ultrasound scan: greater than twelve follicles or large ovaries less than 10 ml (0.4 oz) in volume.
- Irregular ovulation or no ovulation: < six to nine periods per year.
- Excess male hormones called hyperandrogenism, either by observation (acne or excess hair) or the presence of high blood testosterone.

PCOS is probably the most common of female fertility problems. It essentially means there is either no ovulation or infrequent ovulation.

If a woman is ovulating well she produces an egg around twelve times in twelve months. If a woman is not ovulating at all the pregnancy opportunity rate is zero; you cannot conceive if there is no egg. If a woman ovulates just a couple of times in those twelve months you are very likely to miss the fertile window.

Congenital adrenal hyperplasia

The adrenal gland sits up on the kidney. It makes a lot of hormones, the male-like ones of which are called androgens. If it makes too many of these, ovulation can be affected.

Women affected with congenital adrenal hyperplasia, which is uncommon, have more acne than normal and excess, male-like hair growth. The male-pattern hair effects are beard area hair, pubic and chest hair and loss of scalp hair. Affected women are also particularly good at some sports, which is causing controversy for the International Association of Athletics Federations.

Thyroid disease

The thyroid gland produces thyroxine, a hormone that essentially controls our metabolic rate or how fast our body works. It is more or less the body's accelerator. Too much thyroxine means we metabolise too fast, lose weight and feel exhausted; too little and we slow down and gain weight. There can be fertility effects in women from either too much or too little.

Too little thyroxine can affect ovulation, implantation of the embryo and early pregnancy, as these are high metabolic need situations. Having too little thyroxine is far more common than is having too much.

Other hormonal problems

There are many hormones that may affect fertility. One is prolactin, if it is high. The rare tumour known as a prolactinoma in the pituitary gland may cause this. In one rare condition known as androgen insensitivity syndrome, a person is genetically male but the testosterone does not work at all. People with this condition are born looking very female but at puberty have no periods because they lack a uterus. It is rare.

Sometimes the ovaries run out of eggs early, which is known as premature ovarian insufficiency. Menopause happens young and a female's hormones stop being made.

Hyperinsulinemia, or too much insulin, is a common problem and the leading cause of PCOS. It can be associated with high blood pressure and high cholesterol, and is called metabolic syndrome or syndrome X.

TRAFFIC HAZARD	Hyperinsulinemia and PCOS

This might be an old left-over evolutionary survival syndrome. Insulin acts like a growth hormone and causes a human to store fat. High insulin causes more fat storage during times of food abundance, then when food is scarce the hyperinsulinaemic human has more fat reserves to live on. Hyperinsulinaemic PCOS women gain weight easily and stop ovulating, then when they face famine or food scarcity they lose weight and ovulation is restored. Then they become fertile while the average or skinny women lose fertility. This was a hugely advantageous genetic condition for our cavewomen ancestors. Hyperinsulinemia is also useful for the men as a survival genetic condition.

 ## Weight

If a woman is underweight her levels of female hormones may drop, and she may stop ovulating (there may be an evolutionary advantage to not ovulate during a famine or at times of food deprivation). A simple weight gain of only 5 kg (11 lb) almost always works, as this seems to be the magic amount of weight gain needed to re-establish ovulation.

 ## Endometriosis

Endometriosis is a disease of the endometrium, the tissue that lines the inside of the uterus. In this disease tissue grows outside the uterus in an ectopic place. You may have heard of this disease – 4 per cent of fertile women and 40 per cent of infertile women have it. It can manifest itself in a few ways, but the most common is pelvic pain and particularly period pain.

The theories about why the endometrium grows outside the uterus and causes problems, are many, and we don't know exactly why it occurs.

Just prior to the period starting, women with endometriosis may have spotting, and during the period more pain than normal. The bladder and bowel may be involved as well. The disease is highly inflammatory and inflammatory chemicals seem to affect the local area, making the implantation of the embryo

Prevalence and anatomical distribution of endometriosis

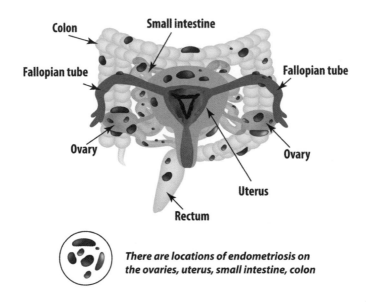

There are locations of endometriosis on the ovaries, uterus, small intestine, colon

more difficult. Also, the endometriosis may cause anatomical effects like scarring, affecting the ability of the ovary to function or the tubes to move.

There seems to be a genetic predisposition to the disease, with age playing a significant role. The older the woman the worse the disease, because it has been in the pelvis longer.

TRAFFIC HAZARD | Case history

I have two interesting stories about how endometriosis can pop up in strange places. A colleague had a patient who often had epileptic fits just prior to her period. She had a CT scan that showed a lesion on her brain. A neurosurgeon removed it – it was endometriosis in her brain. Cured!

Another woman had a left index fingernail that always ached during a period. A small lesion of endometriosis was found under the nail and removed. Once again – cured!

Endometriosis can also present with few if any symptoms although the disease is quite severe. It is a complicated disease that all reproductive doctors know well; the surgery for it is discussed later in the book.

Fallopian tubes

The fallopian tubes are amazing and problems with them are a common cause of infertility, accounting for up to one quarter of cases. In fact, tubal diseases led to the start of IVF. Gynaecologist Dr Patrick Steptoe and physiologist Dr Robert Edwards got together and the rest is history. Englishwoman Louise Brown, the

FALLOPIAN TUBE OBSTRUCTION

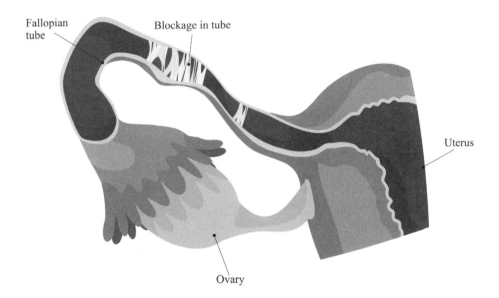

Fallopian tube

Blockage in tube

Uterus

Ovary

world's first IVF baby, had a mother with tubal disease. Tubal disease is one of the most significant causes of female infertility, with a rate as high as 25 per cent.

The role of the fallopian tubes is twofold: they collect the ovulated egg and move it to the distal tubal region called the ampulla. There it awaits any sperm, or it meets sperm that are already waiting there. As you will remember, sperm can survive for days in the fallopian tube.

If fertilisation occurs, then the tiny microscopic embryo will move down the fallopian tube over approximately five days and then move into the uterus, where it will implant.

There are many possible tubal problems.

Pelvic inflammatory disease

Pelvic inflammatory disease (PID) is a common problem and almost always results from a sexually transmitted infection. Chlamydia is the most common, while gonorrhoea is another. Most women will have had at least one pelvic infection in their lifetime, and this may damage the fallopian tubes and cause infertility.

If the fallopian tubes are blocked, the egg and sperm cannot travel along them. The American Center for Disease Control and Prevention (CDC) states that one in eight women who have a history of PID will have fertility issues. If your partner has had PID then investigation may be appropriate before trying to conceive.

 ### Ectopic pregnancy

Your female partner may have had an ectopic pregnancy, where the pregnancy was in the fallopian tube. It may be a random event with no cause but is surprisingly common, occurring in up to 2.5 per cent of normal pregnancies.

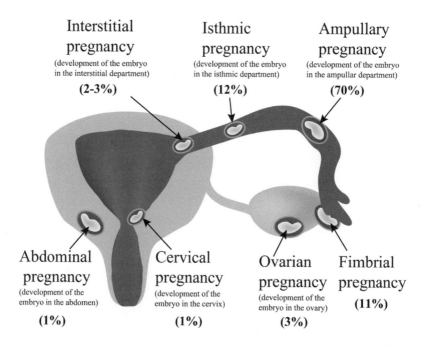

Types of ectopic pregnancy

Interstitial pregnancy
(development of the embryo in the interstitial department)
(2-3%)

Isthmic pregnancy
(development of the embryo in the isthmic department)
(12%)

Ampullary pregnancy
(development of the embryo in the ampullar department)
(70%)

Abdominal pregnancy
(development of the embryo in the abdomen)
(1%)

Cervical pregnancy
(development of the embryo in the cervix)
(1%)

Ovarian pregnancy
(development of the embryo in the ovary)
(3%)

Fimbrial pregnancy
(11%)

If previous PID has scarred the tubes enough to be the cause the rate climbs to 25 per cent or more.

If one tube has been removed because of a previous ectopic pregnancy the other tube may have problems and fertility may be reduced or not possible due to obstruction and blockage.

 ## Pelvic abnormalities

A lot can go wrong in a pelvis that will affect the reproductive potential of a woman, including fibroids, adenomyosis and adhesions.

UTERINE FIBROIDS

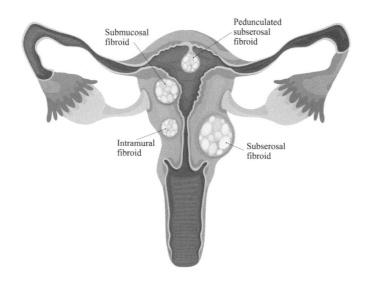

A **fibroid** is a benign growth in the uterine wall that can affect fertility. Think of it as a benign tumour that looks like a knot in the wood of a tree. It is a solid mass that ranges in size from small (less than 1 cm/0.4 in) to huge. Fibroids that bulge into the uterine cavity of the uterus are the most significant: they may compress the small tunnel where the fallopian tube enters the uterus, effectively blocking it.

Very rarely a fibroid is malignant; the ratio is approximately one in every nine hundred fibroids. These are called leiomyosarcomas. Benign fibroids do not turn malignant; the malignant ones were cancerous from the start. Unfortunately, they can be hard to tell apart.

Adenomyosis causes the uterine wall to thicken up, with the cells in the endometrium effectively invading the uterine wall. Periods become heavier and more painful and the uterine wall enlarges, obstructing the small fallopian tube. I call it a uterine wall version of endometriosis and the symptoms can be similar.

This condition tends to be more associated with older women and is rarely seen in the young. Its actual effect on fertility is harder to prove but is suspected. The best surgery for symptomatic women with a big adenomyotic uterus is a hysterectomy after fertility is no longer required.

Scar tissue in the pelvis is known as **adhesions**. These can be caused by a multitude of reasons and they distort normal anatomy. The ovary may be stuck fast away from the tube. The tube may be scarred and non-functional. The bowel may be adhering to the uterus, ovary and tubes.

Adhesions around the uterus

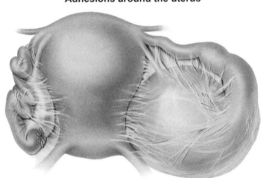

Previous surgery can lead to adhesions. Generally, good surgery with excellent surgical technique reduces adhesions, however, significant bleeding after the procedure or an infection can create scarring. Foreign material also sometimes causes adhesions. Laparoscopic (keyhole) surgery appears to result in less scar formation than open surgery (through an open incision).

A ruptured appendix or an abscess can cause terrible adhesion formation due to peritonitis, or infection of the peritoneum.

Adhesions within the uterus can occur after curettes or infections. This is called Asherman's syndrome.

Sexual dysfunction

Difficulties in having sex are not uncommon but are rarely discussed. The most common is a condition called vaginismus, an involuntary spasm of the vaginal

TRAFFIC HAZARD	Sex therapy

- Sometimes a lack of sex is the only cause of infertility. At other times the sex problems are only part of the fertility problem.
- Sex therapists are experts, and in my experience have excellent success rates at treating sexual dysfunction. They can help almost every couple.
- Men rarely want to go to a sex therapist appointment, but they need to. Couples must be seen together. Your sex life is like your car: if it is not firing on all cylinders or not firing at all it needs a service.
- If you have problems with your sexual relationship go and see a sex therapist.

muscles that essentially prevents penetration by the penis. The muscles can be very strong.

What sets up this situation can vary. Various causes such as sexual trauma in the past may have started it. Pelvic pain such as endometriosis may cause pain on intercourse.

It can be treated successfully.

Medication

Many medications can affect fertility in women. These can be over-the-counter medications, prescription medications and, sometimes, recreational drugs.

Some affect ovulation, such as non-steroidal anti-inflammatory drugs or some psychiatric drugs. Some affect the endometrium; some, like many antidepressants, the libido. Some may be embryo toxic, that is, they may damage an embryo, and are best avoided.

Most prescription medications have a grading system regarding their risk to a pregnancy. The grades are A, B, C, D then X. For example, antibiotics like amoxicillin are grade A, totally safe, and the same with paracetamol, while X is dangerous to the foetus. Thalidomide would today be an X. Roaccutane for acne is an X. If you are trying for a pregnancy you should check any medication you wish or need to take with your pharmacist or doctor with regard to fertility and pregnancy issues.

 ## Congenital malformations

There are a lot of possibilities, but we'll begin with Müllerian anomalies. These are developmental mistakes in the reproductive organs.

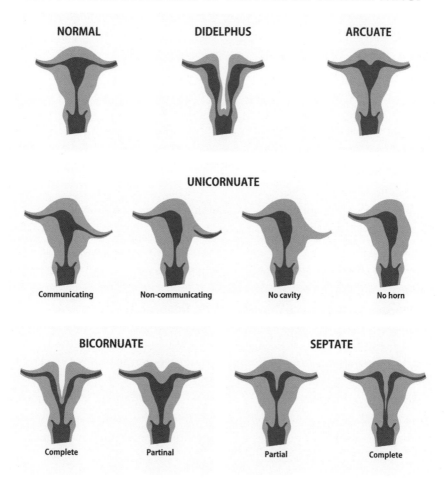

CONGENITAL ANOMALIES OF THE FEMALE GENITAL TRACT

Müllerian anomalies include the following:

* The lack of a vagina, tubes, cervix or uterus. The lack of a uterus is the most common.

- Half a uterus: in normal development two tubes grow down and fuse together to form one tube. Here only one tube forms.
- Two uteruses: with this there are two tubes but no fusing. It can even involve duplication of the uterus, cervix and vagina.

There are other anomalies, some of which cause infertility and others that may reduce fertility or contribute to miscarriage or pregnancy issues. Discuss any congenital malformations with a specialist gynaecologist.

 ## Unexplained infertility

A large proportion of infertility unfortunately remains unexplained – the initial standard tests do not explain the cause. There are a lot more tests a couple can have and many different opinions as to how to manage the infertility from this point onward.

Some specialists advocate that if no abnormal test result is found on basic testing, which includes a tubal dye test, ovulation test and a semen analysis, then depending on their age the couple should simply keep trying naturally. Up to 35 per cent will conceive over two years with no treatment, potentially more if the couple is younger.

For couples where the woman is aged thirty-five or over, IVF becomes useful as the time to pregnancy is quickest and it offers the chance to freeze embryos. This is important.

For older couples, if you use a freeze-all-embryos approach to the first few cycles (with good ovarian reserve and good embryo quality) and aim to freeze, say, four embryos, then in three years or so you can use these embryos to potentially conceive. The pregnancy chance of an embryo is related to the age of the female, not when the embryo is transferred back to the uterus. That is, freezing an embryo locks in the potential of the female age at the time of freezing.

In Australia, and many other countries where IVF costs are low, this freeze-all approach to build up some embryos first is financially achievable and, in my opinion, a good option.

 ## Get involved, guys

There is recent, strong evidence to show that couples with infertility who are actively involved in decision making do better than those who take a more passive approach and let the doctor's dictate treatment.

Get informed and involved; reading this book is an excellent step!

TRAFFIC HAZARD	Summary

The female factors that affect fertility are many; they include:

- ovulation disorders such as PCOS
- hormonal disorders such as thyroid, prolactin or excess male hormone
- fallopian tubal disorders due to sexually transmitted infections
- sexual dysfunction, often due to endometriosis or previous trauma
- anatomical problems, from congenital to those acquired due to diseases
- being under- or overweight and lifestyle issues
- the unexplained, when no obvious answers are found from basic tests

CHAPTER 10

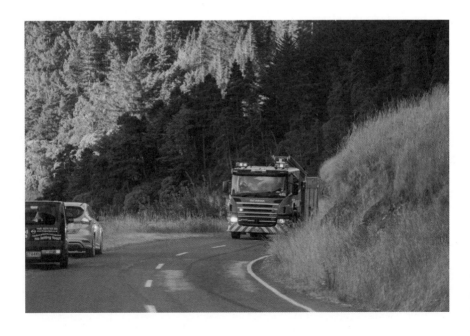

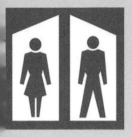

Getting help

TRAFFIC HAZARD

If after twelve months of trying that pregnancy test remains negative, it's time to take the step that one in six couples must take if they want to pursue the idea of having a baby: seek help.

This chapter will outline in extensive detail what goes on at that first visit and in particular why. There is quite a lot involved in that first visit to the specialist and I trust that by the end of this chapter you will have a very clear understanding.

 ## Your general practitioner

The first step for the majority is to go to their general practitioner. For those couples who have already had a child or a previous pregnancy that should be after six months, not twelve. That's a simple but almost entirely unknown fact for most couples and it's worrying how few know this. During 2000 I worked in Dublin, Ireland. The average delay before seeing a fertility specialist was four and a half years. That is a lot of heartache.

Your GP is the first point of contact. They will take a history and either offer advice or refer you on to a fertility specialist.

Infertility specialist

This is where I arrive on the scene. In Australia and many other countries infertility specialists are generally gynaecologists with an interest or further training in infertility. The sub-specialty is called reproductive endocrinology and infertility (REI). It requires further years of training.

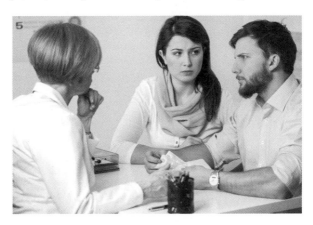

REI extra training covers the entire spectrum of infertility and male and female reproductive hormones. There are a few specialists, known as andrologists, who deal with male hormone issues only.

At the first consultation the couple are seen together. *This is vital*. Men often want to be absent from this first consult but you both need to attend.

 Both partners, male and female, should attend the first specialist visit.

Male factors make up 30 to 40 per cent of the causes of infertility, and up to 40 to 50 per cent if IVF is needed. Often there is more than one cause, as about 70 per cent of the time couples share the reasons for the infertility. Either way the doctor needs to see you both.

TRAFFIC HAZARD	Adam's story: The fear of failure

I nursed my wife through two operations to restore her fertility.

She had one ovary only, which was polycystic, and we had been told months earlier that she was infertile with endometriosis. After the second surgery we sat in our doctor's office eagerly awaiting the news on how the surgery went and what our prospects of her falling pregnant were. After being given encouraging news of a positive outlook ahead I was suddenly told it was my turn.

What? I had not even thought about me in the equation yet – it had all been focused on my wife, her one polycystic ovary and the fear that it would never produce an egg. Of course, it takes two, and it had to be determined if I was the problem. Within minutes a pathology form for a semen analysis was in my hand and I was about to face the biggest test of my life.

I had never failed anything in my life. In obtaining my professional qualifications I had been quite successful in my studies. School, a degree and four post-graduate courses later and I had never ever failed an exam. My immediate macho reaction was: 'I am not about to fail a test now!'

The two-day wait for the pathology gave me time to consider the enormity of this test. You can re-sit an exam, but I did not see a sperm test as being something that you could re-sit or study harder for the next time. After all my wife had gone through I didn't want to let the team down now.

Friends of ours had tried for five years to fall pregnant. Even the closest of friends do not discuss the details of treatment, but as far as I knew it did involve both of them. For the man it involved a 'needle in the nuts', and for the woman a lot of heartbreak and anguish. The road ahead seemed an extremely daunting one.

(Cont.)

Our friends' success and their positive support – if they could do it anyone could – combined with the assertive confidence of our doctor gave us direction. His statement that he would get us a child gave us hope. First, I had to pass the most important test of my life.

I think every thirty-year-old male has doubts over his ability to father a child. Do I work? Am I shooting blanks? Will I do my job? Suddenly, nothing else matters and your role is the most important thing you have ever done in your life.

Luckily, I passed the test! Four months later we fell pregnant and I am now the proud father of a gorgeous little boy. According to our doctor there was never any doubt.

The confidence of your doctor and your confidence in his or her ability are key ingredients in making the whole process more relaxing and stress free – which I believe makes all the difference.

The first consultation is often nerve-racking but the best thing to do is to think about it before you go. The doctor will want to know a lot about both of you. Do a little homework; look back over your life to date. Were there any operations when you were young? Did you have any illnesses like mumps? Any admissions to hospital? Find out a little about the family history. Maybe there is infertility in the family, maybe someone had multiple miscarriages. Perhaps Uncle John has no children for a reason, or just one after ten years of trying. It might involve discussing this with your parents, and that's not always easy.

It's also a good idea to have a clear and honest discussion with your partner. Many couples have past experiences they conceal from the other partner that might be helpful to a doctor, such as a termination of pregnancy when they were younger, or his former girlfriend had a termination or a sexually transmitted infection. Such information can help the doctor greatly but, obviously, it can be a difficult topic to bring up with a partner.

However, finding out information like this about one's partner in a doctor's office is a lot more stressful and difficult than it is at home, in a private environment and circumstance.

TRAFFIC HAZARD — Don't be an ostrich

Once in my office a man revealed that he had two children from a previous marriage to his totally unaware current wife of ten years. He was paying maintenance for both and had been for years. I decided to leave the couple alone for fifteen minutes to see if they would carry on with the consult. When I came back to the room the temperature was positively frigid!

The head-in-the-sand approach is one that can have some awkward results. It is far better to bring these issues up sooner rather than later, and in private.

It's also important to understand the doctor's perspective on much of this information. We are not there to make moral judgements. Patients might be horribly embarrassed to admit to a termination or to multiple previous partners, to STDs, or even to admit to previous sexual abuse. But it doesn't affect how the doctor treats them. It shouldn't, and it doesn't. As professionals, doctors have a duty of care to help their patients. The information patients give is important and it can be extremely sensitive; doctors will treat it accordingly and their patients professionally, have no doubt of that. That goes for practice staff as well.

Finally, everybody should be treated equally. If the prime minister or president and their partner come to see a doctor, they will be treated the same. If they smoke, they will tell them to stop. If they are overweight, they get no special treatment. Infertility does not discriminate based on social status and nor do doctors.

Male history

At the first consultation the doctor will take a history from both of you and probably examine you both.

For men, there are several questions:

- How long have you been trying? How many months or years?
- Have you had any previous pregnancies – children, terminations, miscarriages, ectopic or even just a positive pregnancy IVF cycle that was over quickly?

- Have you had any previous pregnancies with other partners? This can be tricky sometimes. If you are nervous about this question you can tell the doctor separately when being examined. Admitting to having two children with a previous partner to your current partner now can be seriously awkward. Obviously, this holds for both men and women.
- Have you had a sperm count done yet? Some men have already had one done by the GP. Make sure you bring it or arrange for any results to be available at the consultation. The sex bit is usually not an issue, but the sperm count is. A normal sperm count pretty much lets the guy off the hook. An abnormal one may or may not be a serious issue depending on the extent of the problem.
- Do you have any sex problems? How often are you having sex, and in which part of the female cycle? Do you have any issues with impotence, low libido or infrequent sex? There are a lot of busy couples having infrequent sex. This is something men just do not like to talk about with others and most couples are less than open on this matter. It is obviously important.
- Do you have any previous reproductive issues – impotence, STDs, low sperm counts or evaluations? I often ask the same question in different ways. One of the most obvious differences between men and women is in verbal honesty or openness. Men are very reluctant to share about themselves, while usually women will give it all. From a doctor's point of view women provide a full history, but getting information from some men can be like pulling teeth.

I once examined a man and noted that his left testicle was missing and his right one was small and in the groin. I asked him why he never mentioned that in the history about himself. Men are not forthcoming about reproductive matters.

My advice to men is: hide nothing in the consultation. If you are nervous about sharing, arrange to tell the doctor alone, but do tell him or her.

There are a few things we really need to know about.

Mumps. Telling your doctor you had mumps is a must, particularly if this happened in puberty or adolescence and even more so if the mumps spread to the testes.

Late puberty. Was your puberty delayed compared to that of other teenagers? Some simple questions can help if you are not sure. For example, how often do you shave? Most men shave daily but a few men with low hormone levels shave once a week or so. They may have poor muscle development, they may feel weak compared to other men, and their genitalia may be smaller.

History of illness. Your doctor will want to know of any illnesses you have had or currently have, such as a head injury, diabetes and asthma – the list is long. Don't forget anything, however small.

History of surgery. Check with your parents if you're not sure of your surgical history. Important issues include previous hernia repairs as a child, which can damage the vas deferens, and, particularly, undescended testes that were brought down.

Occupation and environment. The important thing here is exposure to substances or situations that are toxic for the testes. These include exposure to heat in a boiler room at 50°C (122°F), radiation, heavy metals such as lead or cadmium, pesticides, working in a nuclear reactor or doing mobile phone tower repairs. I had one patient who worked with printing inks, which affected his sperm count.

Drug use. Here it's best to be honest. Marijuana is a big one, but anabolic steroids for bodybuilding are another. The common ones are alcohol and tobacco. Studies show clearly that patients underestimate their drinking and smoking by as much as 30 per cent.

Medication. Medical drugs can affect semen, most obviously chemotherapy drugs along with medications used for gastritis and some antibiotics such as tetracyclines.

Family history. There are conditions that occur in families: there might be other cases of infertility, recurrent miscarriages (three or more) or a child with a medical condition. There is quite a list. Mention any cancers, as a few of these can have a genetic basis. Don't worry too much if you are not sure, as the doctor is trained to know the questions to ask. Essentially, we are medical detectives.

 Examination

Your doctor will perform a brief examination of the male, usually beginning with an examination of the reproductive organs, the penis and testes. For men this is a new thing. They don't have regular Pap smears of the cervix. Rarely has any of this area been examined.

Almost all my male patients are quite anxious about this and they look like they're thinking I might bite them. Rest assured, doctors rarely bite patients nowadays.

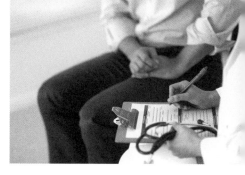

I think many men worry that I might comment on the size of their penis, but I don't. I've seen a few thousand, both large and small, but a doctor's office isn't going to be a place where a penis is at its best.

The examination will include the following:

- Penis examination, to check size and the opening at the end called the meatus.
- Testes examination, particularly to check that both are descended into the scrotum and for size and consistency. They should be of equal size, and usually the left hangs a little lower. Rarely does a lump show up, which might mean testicular cancer – the highest risk is in men with undescended testes not brought down until later in life.
- Examination of the vas deferens and epididymis. The vas feels like a hard cord on the scrotum, on both sides of the scrotum. Men with CBAVD have none.
- A check for a varicocele (the varicose vein in the testes). Often a cough will show it.
- Secondary sexual characteristics, like muscle mass, body shape and distribution of hair.
- Sometimes the doctor might look for other specific things, from breast examination for gynaecomastia (enlargement) through to visual field testing (if a prolactin tumour is suspected) and, rarely, a rectal examination of the prostate. This involves a palpation of the prostate with a finger per the rectum.
- A general weight and blood pressure check might also be done. Morbid obesity deserves some medical attention. If the male is aged forty or over I send him to his GP for a full medical called the 'pre-dad' medical. I'm aiming to make the male a dad and want him in great shape.

Most examinations of men are quick and usually little is found. It is not a bad idea to check yourself out first to discover any problems.

Female history

Men shouldn't complain too much about being examined or the semen test – they get the easy end of infertility.

For the woman there is a lot more to do, and consequently doctors need to organise tests in many areas. These include the menstrual cycle to confirm ovulation, the fallopian tubes, the anatomy of the reproductive organs (usually by ultrasound), maybe a hysteroscopy and laparoscopy (keyhole surgery), and a lot of blood tests. Add to that pre-conception Pap smears and breast lump checks. It is recommended that folate tablets be taken for at least three months prior to conception.

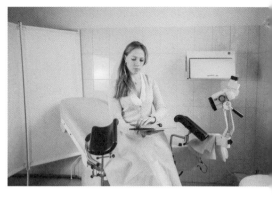

Taking a woman's medical history is like taking a man's, but there are a few differences.

Age and time attempting to conceive. A woman's age is incredibly important, as it affects the way an infertility specialist will approach the couple's issues. We might direct them into assisted reproductive techniques (ART) rather than a more conservative approach of waiting a little longer. The same applies regarding the time a couple has been trying to conceive. If a couple has been trying for four years the percentage chance per month is low, at 1 per cent, compared to six months of trying.

Previous pregnancies and outcomes. This includes live births, miscarriages, ectopic pregnancies and terminations.

Sometimes women will be more comfortable telling you of a termination when you are examining them separately from their partner. If they conceived easily with a previous partner and not with this partner it raises suspicions about the male, particularly if his history includes no previous pregnancies with a previous partner.

Sex frequency and any problems. Couples find this question awkward, but they shouldn't. It is amazing how often the lack of regular sex at the ovulatory time is to blame for reduced fertility. A couple I saw while working at the Hammersmith IVF unit in London were both rather busy. I asked them to get out their extensive diaries and work out past dates of ovulation and sex. They had only had two opportunities to conceive in the previous twelve months!

Pain on intercourse can mean endometriosis or a sexual dysfunction that needs addressing. Sometimes no penetrative sex is ever actually happening.

Menstrual cycle length and period pain. A menstrual cycle shorter than twenty-one days or longer than thirty-five days is uncommon and almost always anovulatory, meaning not producing an egg. Cycle length does change, surprisingly, and even an occasional missed period causes concern. After years on the pill (and more years now that women are leaving children until later) the variation from the regular twenty-eight-day cycle worries women. It probably shouldn't. Period pain is often normal but excessive pain can be linked to endometriosis.

Current gynaecological symptoms. These include breast milk, menstrual pain, abnormal bleeding during a cycle such as mid-cycle bleeding or premenstrual bleeding. Post-coital bleeding (PCB) is a major concern and the cervix must be reviewed by the specialist to exclude any abnormality, particularly early cervical cancer. A lot of women on the pill have PCB due to hormonal effects, but women trying to conceive are not on the pill. Weight gain, hair growth (called hirsutism) and pimples are often linked to polycystic ovarian syndrome. Tiredness is sometimes due to anaemia or hypothyroidism. It's a long list.

Surgery history and complications. This includes previous appendicitis, bowel surgery and hernia repairs. It is surprising, given the amount of internal anatomy women have, that the risks from surgery are not recognised. Adhesions may occur after a ruptured appendix and such events would be a significant risk factor for future fertility. Major bowel surgery for colitis or Crohn's disease should be reported. Of note here is childhood surgery in the pelvis, which is often forgotten. If possible, check with your parents before the initial consultation to make sure you have not missed anything in your medical history.

Past and current medical history. This is also a large list, but diseases like diabetes, thyroid disease, hypertension, arthritis, anorexia and so on come to mind. Many illnesses can impact on fertility. It's not smart to conceive if you are in poor health or a medical condition is not under control, as there may be pregnancy problems. I am still a practising obstetrician, in fact, most of the infertility couples who come to me return for pregnancy care if they are successful. It is in my interest, and more so the interest of the patient, to optimise health before a pregnancy, including pre-pregnancy investigation for Rubella status and making sure they have started taking folate and reduced or stopped smoking and so on.

Past gynaecological history. Sexually transmitted infections (STIs) are still common and the more partners one has had the greater the risk. Often STIs are silent and tubal damage may have occurred without any signs. Chlamydia is still around, as are herpes, gonorrhoea (rarely) and, even less often, syphilis.

It is important to know about previous cervical surgery for an abnormal Pap smear, as the cervix may be affected and scarred. It is difficult to elicit on a first visit to a new specialist, but rape, sexual abuse and sexual trauma may have an influence on a woman's fertility.

Recent Pap smears. It is important for a woman to have had a recent Pap smear. If she has not, a cervical abnormality may go unchecked. If the woman conceives she will easily delay her next Pap smear for at least a year. Previous treatment such as diathermy to the cervix or a cone biopsy may affect the cervix. Bring a copy of the most recent Pap smear result or have the GP send it with the referral letter.

Current medications and drug and alcohol use. Medications are rated regarding safety, as explained earlier. Alcohol, tobacco and recreational drugs have also been addressed. The difference between men and women is that women can get pregnant and carry a foetus for nine months. Drugs, alcohol, tobacco and recreational drugs can affect a pregnancy and a foetus. Think about it from the perspective of the foetus.

Recreational activities. It's less common for a woman's occupation to affect her fertility. Social activities might include excessive exercise, which can affect ovulation.

Family history. Taking a family history may point to an area of fertility interest. Recurrent miscarriages, infertility in relatives, early menopause, diabetes or cancer may be relevant. Genetic problems in the family such as cystic fibrosis or a child with a disability may be important. Sometimes it is worth asking your parents questions about the wider family.

 Examination

Examination of the woman consists of a general examination for hirsutism (excess hair), pimples (both signs of PCOS) and sometimes blood pressure. A breast examination (with an aging reproductive population these become relevant) and a Pap smear should be performed, if not recently done. Weight and height are measured to calculate BMI. There will be an abdominal examination, followed by a pelvic examination which may show tenderness, indicating ovarian cysts or other abnormalities. A vaginal ultrasound scan at the doctor's rooms or elsewhere may pick up abnormalities, cysts, anatomical malformations, swollen infected tubes or abnormal ovaries with PCOS.

At this point the doctor will have a lot of information and be formulating an approach. They might even suggest some counselling if it appears to be necessary, or request another specialist to review current medical conditions such as diabetes.

ROUGH SURFACE	Summary

- If infertility is affecting your relationship you need to get help after just six to twelve months of trying to fall pregnant.
- Start with your general practitioner then consult a specialist who deals with infertility. REI sub-specialists have done advanced training in reproductive medicine.
- The consultation will involve both of you, which is important as men are a significant factor in the infertility equation.
- Before you seek help and go to that consultation, do some homework on yourself. Get all the important information you can.
- Both of you will be questioned, then examined.
- Be honest. Expect some very personal questions: it's the only way we can help you.
- Rule number one is to *get help*!

CHAPTER 11

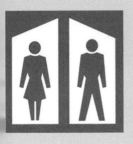

Pinpointing his problem

E ach doctor has slightly different ways of doing things, but just as for a car check-up the basics are common. It all starts with a jar.

 ## Semen analysis

The semen analysis is a test of reproductive potential – no wonder it causes men concern! It can be very confronting. My advice? Get the answer to the question sooner rather than later.

Semen analysis can return results ranging from normal through to azoospermia, meaning no sperm; there are many possible variations. WHO recommends two semen tests at least four

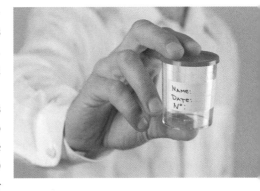

weeks apart, and the routine test is done following approximately three days of abstinence from ejaculation to maintain some consistency across samples.

Sperm counts fluctuate greatly, which is normal. The count can be influenced by many factors including frequency of fevers, which can affect sperm counts for months after the fever, a course of antibiotics, some medications and many other things. Personally, if the semen analysis is normal once I find that acceptable. If abnormal I get a repeat check done four weeks later. Your doctor may request a semen analysis from an accredited laboratory. A sample is required and there are two ways to achieve it – or three if you consider a biopsy of the testes. Let's start with the simple ways.

 Get a semen analysis done at an accredited laboratory.

A sample can be collected in a special sterile container and returned to the lab either directly (because the sample was collected in a special room the lab provides) or it can be brought from home or some other place. The lab will give instructions on how quickly you need to get the sample to the lab.

Most labs have a special sperm collecting room specifically for men and set up accordingly. An appointment is made, and appropriate paperwork filled in. Correct identification of the sample is vital. There may be a cost, and this varies depending on the testing asked for by the doctor.

Sperm collecting rooms vary greatly, from sophisticated facilities to a simple toilet. Most have some literature you can look at or even videos to help arousal. In the London clinic I worked at, a guy came out and mentioned we needed to replace our *Playboy* magazines as he'd read the same ones as a teenager! We sent a male scientist out to buy fresh literature.

Sometimes the female partner can help to get a sample. Either way, getting the sample is the important point. I tell the men to remember all those teenage years and the practice they have done for this day.

The second way to get a semen sample is to wear a special condom during sex and then take this into the lab once ejaculation has occurred. However, normal condoms often contain chemicals that are toxic for sperm, so-called spermicides, to aid in contraception and these might interfere with, or affect the semen analysis.

Many men find the whole business of taking a semen sample quite daunting. A strange room, a booked timeslot and pressure can cause anxiety. What if the sperm count is low? What if the man giving the sample is the cause of the infertility? In some ways it is a test of a man's manhood: no wonder some worry. I often reassure men to put all those teenage training years of producing 'a sample' to good use!

The more difficult way to get a semen sample involves extracting sperm from the testes through either a needle or a biopsy. Some men arrive for the first consultation having had a previous vasectomy; for them, getting sperm may involve the hard way. Other men may have no sperm on ejaculation and the doctor suspects there is an obstruction.

As Hippocrates said three thousand years ago, medicine is about making the diagnosis. Getting a semen analysis is the best way to get on and work out what's right and what might be wrong. A few men refuse to give a sample – the head-in-the-sand mentality or, in Australia, the 'she'll be right' mentality. Good counselling can be effective in this case.

In special circumstances the sample may also be frozen after testing. This may serve as a back-up if the man feels he may struggle to produce a sample on the day of IVF egg collection, for example. It may also be frozen if the male cannot be at the egg collection, being absent for a multitude of reasons such as being in military service or a fly in/fly out miner. Samples can be frozen before cancer treatment, chemotherapy or radiotherapy for use afterwards.

Labs may vary but testing within thirty to sixty minutes is common. If the semen sample has been in the jar for two hours, it is virtually untestable and will give false and misleading results. Keeping the sample warm is also important.

Sperm test results can take a while to be returned, and this can be a time of concern and worry for many men. The great test is done, and waiting is the hardest part.

There will be a repeat visit to the doctor a few weeks after the first visit. In that time other tests may be organised for the male, such as a blood test or maybe an ultrasound of the testes. Obviously the number one test is a semen analysis.

The table below outlines what a semen analysis from a qualified laboratory looks like.

Sample	Semen	Date	Reference range (WHO)
Abstinence	3 days		2–5 days
Round cells	Few	Viscosity normal	
Debris	Normal	pH 7.6	7.2–8.4
Cell clumping	0%		<10%
Semen analysis	**Summary**		
Ejaculate volume	3.7 ml		2.0–6.0 ml
Sperm concentration	7.3million/ml	Oligozoospermia	20–250million/ml
Sperm count	27.01million/ejac	Oligospermia	>60million/ejac
Sperm motility	14% rapid progressive	Unusually low	>25%
	19%progressive	Unusually low	>40%

(Cont.)

Motility index	59/300	Abnormally low	>120
Sperm vitality	90%		>75%
Sperm morphology	0% normal forms	Unusually low	2–6%
Teratozoospermia index	1.82 TZI		<2.00
Antisperm antibody	GAM(%)	Negative	Positive >20% Significant >50%
	IgG%		
	IgA%		
	IgM%		
SCSA			
Date tested			
DNA fragmentation index (DFI)	11%	Excellent DNA integrity	<15% excellent DNA integrity
High green (HDS)	3%	Normal	16–24% good
			25–29% fair
			>29% poor DNA
Trail wash			
Preparation method	Redigrad 45/90%		
Total yield	0.6 million progressive sperm (12%)		
Motility at 37%	67%		
Treatment guideline	Low yield of motile sperm	ICSI	

Semen is **alkaline** to counteract the female's acidic vagina. The alkalinity comes from the prostatic and seminal vesicle fluid. A low **pH**, that is, less than 7.0, might mean an obstruction along the vas deferens or absence of the vesicles.

Volume depends on many factors but obviously the abstinence period accounts for the variation here, which is why three days is recommended to keep consistency between samples. Another cause is incomplete samples: it is tricky ejaculating into a cup, and some training might be required. The condom option for collection can help but is tricky itself, as sometimes there is spillage.

There is a natural variation in sperm **concentration** and count. It can be considerable due to many factors, such as illness, sexual frequency, obstruction and so on. Particularly low concentrations may have a genetic cause – 12 per cent of men with no sperm and 4 per cent of men with a low count have a genetic cause. If you multiply the volumes in millilitres by the concentration you calculate the total sperm count.

Vitality indicates the proportion of live sperm. This is useful if there is low motility. Some sperm have motility issues due to a mechanical problem, but they are alive. Poor motility and low vitality might mean lots of anti-sperm antibodies.

Human males have few normal-shaped sperm – 2 to 6 per cent is considered normal. If the percentage of normal-shaped sperm is less than 2 per cent fertility rates fall. This is referred to as the **morphology** of sperm.

If there are high levels of anti-sperm **antibodies,** then fertility will be affected by reduced motility. Binding may be to the sperm head or tail; head binding is worse.

In a **trial wash**, sperm are put to the test. They must swim up a density gradient of fluid, much as salmon swim upstream. The numbers that get to the top of the stream of fluid give us an idea of how well the sperm are working.

Sometimes there are **other cells** apart from the sperm in the semen, such as white blood cells. This may mean there is an infection and is known as leukospermia, from the word for white cells (leukocytes) and sperm.

Occasionally red blood cells turn up. This is unusual, and men notice it very quickly as being abnormal. It can mean infection or trauma. One patient I treated had taken a taekwondo kick to his 'family jewels' during a competition and had blood in his semen. He also had a hugely swollen pair of testes and the damage done to them significantly reduced his sperm count. It took over two weeks for the testes to settle and the man was in a lot of pain. Testes have an excellent blood and nerve supply – not surprising given their importance – and they don't like being kicked!

There are a lot of other tests that can be performed on a semen sample because semen is more than just sperm. For example, the seminal vesicles produce fructose, a sugar, and absence of fructose usually means absence of the seminal vesicles or could mean an obstruction at a level after the seminal vesicles.

 ## Antibodies

Sometimes there are antibodies found in semen that are hostile to sperm. An antibody is a protein produced by B-cells – a type of white blood cell – which attacks a cell or object that is perceived to be foreign.

Sometimes for men with no sperm in their semen, the sperm can only be evaluated by a **testicular biopsy**. They may have obstructive azoospermia, for which the most obvious cause is a vasectomy, or they may have non-obstructive azoospermia.

Some doctor's get a diagnostic biopsy done purely to make a diagnosis but in other circumstances they may do the biopsy at the time of IVF, and if sperm are found they can be used for the IVF with your partner's collected eggs. I have all men tested for their **karyotype**, in order not to miss any obvious gene issues.

Occasionally with low to no sperm we order a **Y-deletion study**. The test looks at the AZF region of the Y chromosome to see if there are deletions of the genes that code for making sperm.

It can be useful to test men's reproductive **hormones**. If the semen analysis is normal then it is probably not needed, but if the semen test is abnormal this result can help the doctor to determine the cause. We can test FSH, LH, testosterone, prolactin and many more.

The testes also make less-common hormones such as inhibin B. A male with no sperm with a high FSH (the coach hormone yelling at the testes), low testosterone (then high LH as this hormone drives testosterone) and a high inhibin B is virtually assured of having no sperm on a biopsy. A low inhibin B might convince the doctor to try a biopsy. Inhibin B is not a universally accepted test by REI doctors, so be aware of this. In fact, doctor's opinions vary on many investigatory tests.

Other **blood tests** that may be performed include glucose testing for diabetes andbiochemical testing for liver disease and cholesterol, as well as drug screens for recreational drugs. The doctor may order an **ultrasound** scan of the testes and scrotum if on examination of the man the doctor finds a lump in the testes or a large varicose vein called a varicocele. They may find a hernia or a fluid-filled cyst of water called a hydrocele. Rarely, the prostate might be the issue or there is a lack of seminal vesicles. The ultrasound might be done trans-rectally. You were warned.

A medical

Some doctors will send men off for a full medical by their GP, especially from the age of forty. In a way it is an excellent line in the sand to get men to have a proper medical check-up.

ROUGH SURFACE	**Summary**

- There are several investigations that you may have to undergo.
- Semen analysis is the cornerstone; you *really* have to do this. A semen analysis looks at count, motility and shape along with many other things.
- You may need a testicular biopsy.
- There are other tests such as blood tests or ultrasounds that may be required.
- You might get sent for a full medical check up.

CHAPTER 12

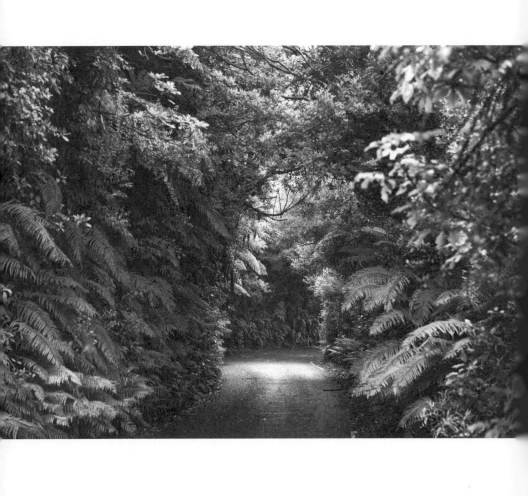

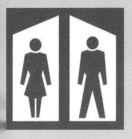

Pinpointing her problem

Tests for females to discover the cause of infertility involve **pre-pregnancy** tests followed by specific **infertility** tests.

Blood tests. I find that most patients prefer as few blood tests as possible, so I try and get as much information as I can from a blood test performed on day three of the menstrual cycle. This is the standard day of the cycle to organise blood tests. The formal blood tests are described in the following pages.

There are four **blood groups**: O, A, B and AB. Then there is the positive or negative factor known as the Rhesus factor.

If a female is a negative blood group and her partner is a positive, there may be issues due to the incompatibility. This is called Rhesus disease and used to be a huge problem. If there were enough anti-D antibodies to attack the baby's blood the baby died inside the mother. The more pregnancies she had, the worse it was. Nothing could be done until blood groups were better understood.

Now we give the mother who is blood group negative an injection at twenty-eight weeks and at thirty-four weeks of anti-D antibodies. This mops up any stray positive foetal blood cells that might have got into her blood from the pregnancy. If she has any small bleeds during the pregnancy, we would give extra anti-D to cover that.

There are a few other **antibodies** labs need to test for in case of a potential blood transfusion down the track. Pregnancy and childbirth is a high-risk time for loss of blood and potentially for blood transfusions. Historically, being pregnant was the single biggest risk to her life a woman could face.

A **full blood count** will be done to check for any anaemias or strange blood conditions such as thalassaemia, which is common in middle Europeans. This test measures the red blood cells, the white blood cells, the platelets (useful in blood clotting) and the haemoglobin.

Testing for **hepatitis B and C** is mandatory in Australia. Hepatitis can be a chronic condition and patients with it are called carriers. The virus lives in the female body permanently, and during pregnancy can cross the placenta to the foetus with significant consequences. If the woman has had a recent case of hepatitis B or C or is a carrier she can be managed appropriately.

Testing for **HIV** is called a screening test and occasionally picks up HIV in a low-risk group. We test all females in Australia (known as universal testing rather than selective testing) so we can better plan a pregnancy if HIV is present. Be aware that false positive tests occasionally occur, that is, the test comes up positive but is found to be false on more accurate testing called a Western blot test.

Most women are vaccinated against **rubella**, also known as German measles, when they are young. With this we check their immunity status: if their antibody levels are absent or low a booster vaccination may be required. Pregnancy must be delayed for twenty-eight days or so depending on the local protocol for vaccinations and safety margins. Rubella is a potentially dangerous infection for the foetus if the mother catches the disease during pregnancy. Like many others, the virus can cross the placenta.

Syphilis is rare but once again is a dangerous disease for the foetus.

Pregnancy requires a decent **iron** intake for both the mother and the foetus. Starting with a good iron level is helpful as iron is the single most important component of haemoglobin, the oxygen-carrying molecule that gives blood its red colour.

Occasionally **B12/folate** levels will be low, and anaemia may result. B12 deficiency anaemia is called pernicious anaemia and requires injections of vitamin B12. Folate is easier to manage as it can be ingested orally.

Vitamin D, which comes from sunshine, is required for bones and teeth and many other processes. A tablet version is now available. Vitamin D has a role in regulating calcium and phosphate levels, and a developing foetus needs it for its own bones and teeth development. As well, low maternal vitamin D may be linked to other diseases in the foetus such as diabetes, multiple sclerosis and even cancer. Fifteen minutes to half an hour in the sun each day is a great way to get sufficient vitamin D.

CMV, **toxo**, **parvo B19** and **varicella** are viral infections. CMV is cytomegalic virus; toxo is toxoplasmosis bacteria; parvo B19 is a virus also known as 'slapped cheek' syndrome or 'fifth' disease; varicella is chicken pox. Previous exposure to infection or a vaccination will protect the mother and in particular the foetus. These illnesses are not really a problem to a woman, but if they cross the placenta and get to the developing foetus they can damage it. Not all IVF units or REI/OBGYN doctors carry out these tests. I do, as I always aim to test the woman with a view to a potential pregnancy.

Low levels of **follicle-stimulating hormone** (FSH) mean something is shutting down the hormones. High levels mean the ovary is not working properly. I think of FSH as a coach who talks to the athlete, the ovary. A poorly performing athlete will make the coach yell louder and consequently the FSH will rise. A low FSH may mean the coach isn't working and so the ovary also does not. It can also mean that the hormone GnRH, which stimulates FSH, is absent.

Luteinising hormone (LH) will ultimately start the actual ovulation process as it suddenly rises. A high level on day three may indicate polycystic ovary syndrome. **Serum LH** tests are a series of blood tests that document the LH surge that causes ovulation; they are very accurate. Often, they are included with ultrasound scanning to document the development of a follicle.

Oestrogen is the main female hormone and is mostly made by the ovary (the athlete). Low levels are seen before puberty and in menopause and in many conditions associated with infertility.

Testing the levels of **anti-Müllerian hormone** (AMH) basically tells you the quantity of eggs in the ovary. It is helpful, but it does not tell you how good the eggs are; it just quantifies the approximate number left.

A **karyotype** test is a genetic test: men are 46XY and females 46XX. There can be variants on this and they can affect fertility. The older test can take a few weeks to get done. Be patient. New modern karyotype tests can be much quicker.

From the pituitary, **thyroid-stimulating hormone** (TSH) drives the thyroid gland to work. Thyroxine hormone is the body's metabolic rate hormone.

Sometimes specific **thyroid** tests are done for thyroxine (made by the thyroid gland) and even anti-thyroid antibodies. High TSH suggests hypothyroidism, when the thyroid is working poorly. Low TSH suggests hyperthyroidism and an over-active thyroid gland.

Prolactin is a pituitary hormone mostly associated with breastfeeding. Small, benign tumours can grow in the pituitary gland in the brain and make this hormone, which affects ovulation. Every textbook mentions it, but I have seen very few high prolactin results due to a prolactinoma in the pituitary gland.

Be warned, this test result can be falsely elevated if there was breast manipulation in the preceding forty-eight hours, thus men should leave their partner's breasts alone before the test.

There are quite a few male-like hormones, or **androgens**, that can be tested for. Obviously, testosterone is the first. The ovary makes some, as does the adrenal gland. Testing for testosterone alone is inaccurate and most labs do a free testosterone level or free androgen index test.

The adrenal androgen blood test looks at dehydroepiandrosterone sulphate as well as androstenedione. If congenital adrenal hyperplasia is suspected, specific tests may be asked for, such as 17-hydroxyprogesterone. Even we REI doctors must get the textbook out to remember how this all works!

A **glucose tolerance plus insulin test** looks for diabetes and insulin resistance. It requires the patient to fast overnight then have a blood test to check her fasting glucose level (and maybe insulin levels, if the doctor wants). The patient then has a drink of glucose. Further blood tests are taken at one hour and two hours to measure glucose and insulin.

Raised **CA125** is commonly linked to endometriosis. It may indicate an ovarian tumour if it is very high, although this is rare. Adenomyosis may also raise it and sometimes it's just up with no good cause.

The hormone **progesterone** is harder to explain but levels go up later in the cycle after a successful ovulation, hence the famous day twenty-one progesterone level test which should be done on the seventh day before the woman's next period. That's day twenty-one if it's a twenty-eight-day cycle, day twenty-seven if it's a longer thirty-four-day cycle and so on. It is basically the cycle length minus seven days.

Ovulation tests

Ovulation tests pinpoint ovulation and confirm it has occurred. Ovulation is a prerequisite to conceiving; it is a cornerstone of fertility. Before IVF came along a woman had to ovulate to conceive.

Many female patients have purchased ovulation kits to confirm if they are ovulating; these can be helpful and test through urine or saliva. They work on

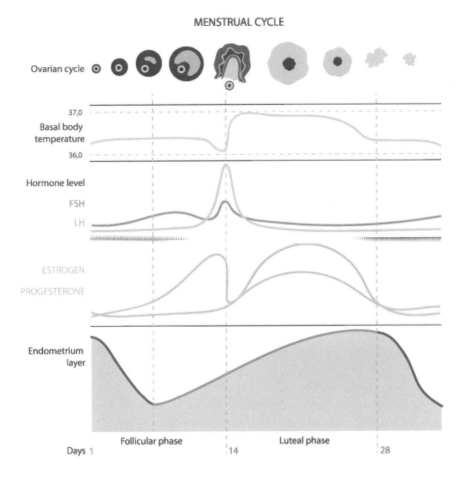

MENSTRUAL CYCLE

the principle of detecting a rise in LH, which is the surge that initiates ovulation. Anovulatory or PCOS patients may have high LH constantly, which can affect the test and give a false positive result.

There is a small but detectable rise in body temperature after ovulation, with the lowest temperature occurring around the actual day of ovulation. The temperature rise of approximately 0.5°C (41°F) can occur from one to five days after the LH surge and therefore up to four days after ovulation, and can show the length of the follicular phase. Tests to measure basal body temperature (BBT) are cheap and relatively simple, but they can be stressful and tiring and not all ovulating women show the classic biphasic (two-phase) rise. Many modern apps on smart phones can help map a woman's menstrual cycle and include instructions on measuring BBT.

Tubal tests

There are three fallopian tube tests: an X-ray hysterosalpingogram, an ultrasound hysterosalpingo-contact-sonography (HYCOSY), or dye can be inserted during a laparoscopy. These tests are important because tubal and pelvic diseases make up to 25 per cent of the causes of infertility.

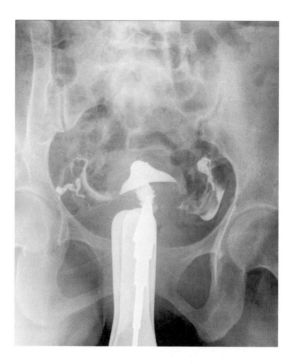

The fallopian tubes are open around mid-cycle and closed later in the cycle, so timing this test is very important. It should be done on days six to ten of the female cycle.

TRAFFIC HAZARD	Day one menstrual cycle

It is vital that this term is understood. The first day of full period bleeding is deemed day one of the female menstrual cycle, and all calculations are based on this. Spotting does not count.

Timing for tests, and ovulation and progesterone and dye studies, are all based on day one of the menstrual cycle.

Ultrasound

Transvaginal (TV) ultrasounds have had an enormous impact on investigation of the infertile female and gynaecology in general. Abdominal ultrasounds are good, but TVs are better. The probe tip is much closer to the organs and tissues the radiologist or gynaecologist wishes to view and therefore provides a better, clearer picture. I'm told it is not uncomfortable (but then, I'll never have one) and takes maybe ten to fifteen minutes. It can assess the uterus, the cavity, the ovaries and the surrounding structures and sometimes it can see tubal disease.

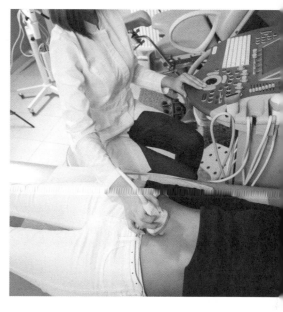

It is important to have the ultrasound scan performed by experienced people. In your town or city there should be a specialised ultrasound unit that only caters for women and is not a general radiology unit. That is the best option. For even more specialised ultrasound, for endometriosis for example, there may be doctors who have great expertise.

Check the unit before you get scans done. Your doctor will be able to help.

Laparoscopy and hysteroscopy

Laparoscopy is an operation that involves inserting a tiny telescope into the pelvis to view the structures. It has been around since the 1960s and is extremely common now, both as a diagnostic tool and for treatment. It offers an excellent view of the pelvis and is very safe.

A diagnostic laparoscopy is a valuable tool to investigate an infertile female. When a laparoscopy is performed with a tubal dye test – injecting dye and watching through the laparoscope – it offers a great deal of information. If a hysteroscopy is added, that is, a look inside the uterus through the cervix, almost all the pelvic reproductive anatomy is directly seen.

Operations take around twenty to thirty minutes and require a full general anaesthetic. They are very safe. If small problems are found they can be fixed during the laparoscopy, but larger problems will be left for another time so that consent can be properly obtained, options fully discussed and scheduling organised.

When considering either a diagnostic or an operative laparoscopy/ hysteroscopy there are two possible types of approach. Some doctors do a diagnostic operation first, that is, a laparoscopy and hysteroscopy. Even if they find diseases like endometriosis or a septum they do not remove it; they take photos and videos and discuss their findings later. I am one of those doctors. I show the female the findings and explain the next step if one is needed.

The second approach is to start the process then to operate and remove disease during the same operation. Many gynaecologists take this approach.

Why do I take the first approach? Because I find I can make an accurate diagnosis in theatre, then plan the next much bigger operation better knowing this. I can explain the next operation more clearly and have in place the appropriate consents for risks, and I can schedule my operative timing more accurately.

Either approach is reasonable.

 ## Other tests

There are several other tests that are sometimes useful in the world of infertility, although they are not commonly used.

Computed tomography (CT) scans are useful to look at any pituitary gland problems in the brain.

During a renal (kidney) CT scan dye is injected into a vein. This is known as an intravenous pyelogram. The scan can track the dye through the kidneys and ureter and then the bladder. It is for structural problems with the ureter (mostly) or the kidneys.

Magnetic resonance imaging (MRI) scans are useful for investigating the pelvis or checking the uterus for fibroids or adenomyosis.

 ## Costs

The costs of more advanced surgery may be an issue that requires discussion. Each country has different funding for medicine. In Australia, there is a fully funded public health system and necessary surgery is free. As well, there is a large private health system with private hospitals, where operations like these will cost the patient depending on health funds and the surgeon's fees.

I suggest you do some research into the surgeon and their costs as there can be quite a range. Make sure you and your partner understand any additional costs, like those for the anaesthetist, health fund excess fees or even instrument costs.

Adding unexpected financial stress to the stress of infertility does not help.

TRAFFIC HAZARD	Saving money

After twelve months of infertility, if your partner has an income, I suggest you both decide to save her income if she plans to take maternity leave. It is in effect bonus money – you two would not have that money if your partner was at home with a baby on maternity leave and without an income stream. I know a few fathers who take the paternity leave option and are stay-at-home dads. The money accumulates and is a huge buffer against any medical costs for infertility treatments, plus you can use it for a holiday if you need a break from the stress of the infertility merry-go-round.

Additional surgical help may also be called on. If the pelvic problem is severe endometriosis, special gynaecological surgeons may be required to do the surgery; it depends on the level of skill of the treating infertility specialist. A bowel surgeon may also be needed if there is bowel involvement and sometimes a urologist is needed as well, to deal with the ureters or bladder. Additional surgeons may add additional costs.

 ## Recovery

It takes a few days to recover from a diagnostic operation and longer if it is more advanced. If surgery cannot be done laparoscopically with the special telescopes, then an open procedure may be required. Recovery from that is much longer – four to six weeks.

 Take time off to care for your partner.

Even some of the simple tests such as hysterosalpingo-contact-sonography to check a woman's tubes are painful so you should always plan on accompanying your partner.

Complications: that's a scary word. Your partner may have a complication during surgery – they do happen, and your doctor is obliged to clearly state the risks.

It's like driving: you try to reduce the risk by driving at the right speed, wearing a seat belt, staying on the correct side of the road and not consuming alcohol. However, all these things cannot reduce the risk to zero and complicated surgery is the same.

ROUGH SURFACE	Summary

Your partner may require many tests for the investigation of infertility. These may vary but cornerstone tests include a day-three hormone profile, an anti-Müllerian hormone level test, a tubal study and ultrasound of the pelvis, and an ovulatory test like the day twenty-one progesterone test. More may be required, along with keyhole surgery. You should understand what these tests are and what information they provide. Keep in mind how much more your partner must do – you probably only had a simple semen analysis. Keep a running log of what's been done and the results, and make sure you know what they mean.

Understand the importance of timing with regard to the test and particularly on which days of your partner's cycle they are done.

Look after your partner during the tests. For surgery, take time off to care for her post-operatively.

CHAPTER 13

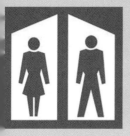

Male infertility treatments

Treatments for the male vary from the simple through to the complex.

 ## The simple options

Let's divide simple up into various areas that make sense:

- *Location*: men must be in the right place for conception to occur.
- *Timing*: they must get the timing right – when ovulation occurs.
- *Age*: they should consider the passing of time and fertility and not leave it too late to start trying to conceive. Age is the main factor in fertility, especially the age of the female.
- *Lifestyle*: both your own and your partner's lifestyle can affect fertility. Tobacco, alcohol, recreational drugs and weight all have an effect.
- *Environment*: heat, cold, the presence of heavy metals and wearing tight clothing can all be factors.
- *Sex*: there is a simple message here: have more!
- *Anatomy*: any problems down there need to be fixed.
- *Medication*: check if they might be the problem.
- *Libido and performance*.

 ## Location

You must be in the right place for fertility to occur. Simply put, you *must* be with your partner when she is ovulating.

Men are often away through work or social activities, or even psychologically absent at the times when they are needed. Australia's economy has changed recently and there is a lot of fly in/fly out work – many men are away at mines, gas fields and so forth. It seems obvious, but if you're not there at the crucial time nothing will happen.

If you feel the urge to have a boys' weekend, try to do this when your partner is not ovulating. It takes two to tango.

Solution: be in the best possible location to help fertility – with your partner when she is ovulating.

Timing

Women ovulate approximately once a month, and the female egg lives for just twenty-four hours. Timing sex for ovulation day is important; if you are away for work or other reasons then your timing isn't right.

The solution can be simple. If you're a fly in/fly out worker and you're out of town at the wrong time your partner's ovulation can be adjusted to coincide with the times when you are home. Easy, especially if your fertility doctor or GP can use medications to move her cycle.

TRAFFIC HAZARD	The fisherman

I had a fisherman patient who was away two weeks out of every four: two on, two off. The trouble was his partner's ovulation occurred when he was away. I put her on a medication called Primolut for two weeks, shifting her ovulation by two weeks, and finally their timing was right. Soon they had 'hooked' a baby.

Timing is vital and being pro-active in this regard will help. The concept of a 'date night' where sex is planned, is well known: busy lives, fewer chances for spontaneity and more life pressures have brought this idea into vogue. Plan a few date nights around ovulation and be pro-active. Your partner will love to know there is something planned and there will be a sense of anticipation. This is always enjoyable.

 Book a date night around ovulation and plan something nice and romantic.

My researched seven-day rule to maximise sperm is more a guideline than a rule. It is unlikely that a sexual frequency and fertility study can be done in humans to work out the best frequency for fertility, but we can extrapolate from animal studies and take a guess.

I tell my patients to have sex each day for seven days and aim to have day five around ovulation. Remember: ovulation roughly occurs fourteen days before the next period. A twenty-eight day cycling female ovulates on day 28 – 14 = day 14. A thirty-two day cycling female ovulates on day 32 – 14 = day 18. My approximate day-five sex on ovulation day allows for the ovulation day to vary, which it does. Female ovulation is not as clockwork as we think; years of follicular tracking by my practice has shown that. If your partner ovulates earlier or a bit later, the seven day regime will catch it and probably also allow some frequent ejaculation time to improve your sperm quality.

| TRAFFIC HAZARD | **The ovulation day rule** |

Cycle length (days) – 14 (days) = ovulation day (approximately).

Imagine your partner's cycle is thirty-one days: 31 — 14 = 17. She is probably ovulating around day seventeen of her cycle.

Start sex about four days before ovulation so ovulation day is around day five of seven days in a row of sex. Even if ovulation varies a bit (and it does), you won't miss it with a seven-day approach.

Have a few days off sex and then have some more as the embryo is trying to implant, as per Professor Sarah Robertson's research showing that semen 'primes' the endometrium of the uterus to help implantation.

I'll leave you to work out the details. Use a calendar or your smart phone app to plan a few months' worth of date nights and add alarms so you don't forget. Remember to show this to your partner. A plan in your head might just stay there and never be articulated. Men don't always say what they think, so you should tell your partner in this case and show her your planning , so that you are both on the same page.

If you have been trying for a year or two to conceive it's probable that sex is becoming a difficult chore. Just do the best you can. Viagra can help and just having it available can relieve men's concerns about performance enough to not need to use it.

Solution: get the timing right.

Age

The single greatest factor affecting a couple's fertility is age, that of both you and your partner. As your partner's eggs age they will lose fertility potential, and as you age there will be consequences.

People are forming relationships later in many Western societies, and your partner's biological clock is running. It's often said that forty is the new thirty, but her ovaries and eggs haven't been told!

 Forty may be the new thirty but no one told the eggs that!

This is a serious matter for you both. Discuss it early in your relationship if age is an issue, if your partner is over thirty. If she is over thirty-five then the topic needs to be considered very soon. If she is aged over forty a frank discussion will save a lot of heartache later.

Prepare for this conversation: bounce your views off someone independent before discussing this with your partner. You may not be sure why you feel the way you do and a session with someone else can really help you understand yourself. Explaining your position to someone else can also help to clarify your thinking. Being noncommittal or vague is not helpful; if you feel like that, work out why and deal with it. Factor in lifestyle and career options as well as age.

You might start the conversation with your partner like this: 'I've thought about having kids at some stage. I've always been keen to be a dad with two kids. I've found the woman I want to have children with, you, and I'd like to have them earlier rather than later. What do you think about when to have them?'

Solution: consider this issue carefully and canvass all the options with your partner. Maximise your fertility window and don't leave trying for children too late. If you start a new relationship with an older partner and children are on the agenda, discuss age and fertility early.

Lifestyle

Having a good lifestyle is important for fertility, with the most important lifestyle changes being quitting smoking, losing weight and reducing alcohol consumption. If you are using recreational drugs like marijuana, stop using them. Obviously, the taking of drugs such as anabolic steroids used at the gym also needs to stop. Take a good long look at your lifestyle and remove anything that could affect fertility.

Both partners need to change but any psychologist will tell you the only person you can change in a relationship is *you*. Start with yourself and your partner will follow.

In my experience the female partner is often making lifestyle changes while the male partner is not. You might really enjoy a big night out with the lads and those binges are a big part of your social life. If you're struggling to have children, make a lifestyle change now.

Weight is important, more so for females but also for males. Overweight men have reduced fertility.

Remember that changes like stopping smoking or weight reduction will bring permanent and proven health benefits and make you a long-term father.

Solution: address lifestyle issues. Changes can make significant improvements to fertility.

 Lifestyle changes will have fertility and long-term health benefits for you both, and your children.

 ## Environment

The effects of environment on men are significant. Sperm grow in a scrotum at a nice 32°C (89.6°F), not the 37°C (98.6°F) of the torso. Heating up the scrotum by wearing tight clothing or exposing it to a hot working environment such as a coal mine may result in your sperm declining in number and motility. A cook near a hot stove provides a classic textbook example of suffering from heat effects. Petroleum products and some associated heavy metals can affect sperm by increasing free radical damage.

Solution: check your sperm count. If you're being affected, seek help. If not, great!

 ## Sex

The message here is simple – have *more* if you can, around ovulation.

As noted earlier in this book, animal and a few human studies show higher breeding rates when there is more sexual frequency. Abstaining prior to ovulation to build up a good sperm count is a bad idea, as studies show that the effects on semen are negative. If abstaining makes sperm DNA damage worse and reduces motility the opposite might be true.

Solution: have more sex around ovulation.

 ## Anatomy

You should check your scrotum and the contents regularly. Is everything in place, does it all function properly? The men I examine for fertility in my examination room have almost never been examined there. I find hernias, varicoceles, hydroceles, cysts, small testes, undescended testes and absent testes.

The best place to examine your man bits is in the shower. Check them out, and if there is something wrong or missing go and see your doctor.

Solution: check out your man bits.

 ## Medication

There are many medications that may affect sperm and its function and many men in older age groups wanting to have children who are taking medication. Common ones include anti-depressants such as Prozac and Zoloft. These can affect libido. Codeine and codeine-like opiate medications can dramatically reduce your sperm count. Some anti-inflammatory drugs can also, especially those called COX-2 inhibitors like Mobic or even simple NSAIDS like Nurofen or Voltaren.

It may seem obvious, but if you are trying to have kids consider the medications you are on or have been on. Even some antibiotics can have temporary effects on sperm count. Some of the early medications for gastritis such as Cimetidine can affect the sperm count. Many chemotherapy drugs will have profound effects, some permanently.

Solution: discuss your medications with your own doctor or a pharmacist and how they may affect fertility.

 ## Libido and performance

Severe stress, poor sleep and physical and mental problems can all decrease your libido. Almost all men have had a performance issue at some stage, but for most it is brief and soon passes. Long-term infertility can have a profound effect on the male and in my experience almost always does.

Solution: address the potential causes of low libido. If there is no improvement, consult your GP.

The complex options

The preceding section dealt with those things a man could fix himself. This section deals with more complex treatments that require some medical intervention, such as IVF and surgery.

Fertility questions are not an easy topic of discussion and most men find that it's quite hard to get their heads around and understand and then to agree to complex treatments. However, you will see that it's all about getting sperm and delivering sperm.

 ## IVF for sperm problems

Simply put, a complex sperm problem occurs when there are either not enough to start a pregnancy naturally or they have poor motility or shape, or perhaps even the sperm DNA is a problem. *See* Chapter 4 for more detail. Sperm may also be absent, that is, azoospermia. This is the ultimate complex problem.

Whatever the issue with the male semen sample the answer will probably be IVF once correctable problems, such as lifestyle or the taking of drugs or medications, are corrected but the problem persists.

IVF is the go-to treatment for this problem, except if there are no sperm. That might require a testicular biopsy; if sperm are found then an IVF will be needed. This is covered in more detail in Chapter 15. Intracytoplasmic sperm injection (ICSI), an additional part of an IVF treatment cycle, is the technique of injecting a single sperm into the egg using microscopes and micro manipulation.

TRAFFIC HAZARD	Intracytoplasmic sperm injection

IVF using ICSI is the single most common and most successful treatment in the world for male factor infertility where the sperm is the issue.

IVF revolutionised the world of infertility in 1978, then intra-cytoplasmic sperm injection revolutionised the IVF world in 1991 when it was finally discovered.

 ## Vasectomy reversal

There has been a great change in relationships over the last century and more people are leaving one relationship for another. During their first relationship, many men decide they have finished making children and for various reasons choose a vasectomy as a permanent form of contraception. If those men form another relationship and decide they want more children with their new partner, there's an obvious problem. Vasectomy reversal is a proven method of restoring natural fertility to men who want to have more children.

 New Zealand leads the world in vasectomies – an estimated 57 per cent of men aged forty to forty-nine have had a vasectomy.

One large follow-up study showed that the two factors that most affected reversal success are the time since the vasectomy was performed and the age of the current female partner. Second relationships tend to be between older couples and age affects the fertility results. Say you have a marriage, two kids and a vasectomy and then separate a few years later. You start a new relationship at age forty with a woman who is around the same age and has her own children. You and your new partner are not in the same situation as a younger infertile couple.

In terms of the operation, patency rates (that is, an open tube with sperm passing through because of the operation) are up to 90 per cent in some centres. Of these men, around 30 to 75 per cent will achieve a pregnancy and a child.

 Overall success rates for a live birth after vasectomy reversal are around 50 per cent.

The results are nowhere near 100 per cent, but few fertility treatments are. Given your circumstances, you and your partner might accept a 30 per cent chance of pregnancy from a vasectomy reversal and let fate decide. You might not feel the same urgency to have children, having already had some. I've done a few vasectomy reversals where the couple was happy to accept the outcome whether it worked or not. Not trying meant they had zero chance. The essential surgical technique to reverse a vasectomy is a tiny repair using a high-powered microscope and excellent surgical technique. You will need a surgeon who has experience with vasectomy reversal and is trained in microsurgical technique, and a hospital that can provide the right support team and equipment.

The surgical reversal is done in one of two ways.

The first method is called a vasovasostomy. The area of the vas deferens that has been blocked is cut and then the two clean ends of the vas sutured together with fine sutures around half as thick as a single human hair.

The second, and technically more difficult, method is called a vasoepididymostomy. With this method the vas is connected to the epididymis. It is truly difficult microsurgery with a lower success rate.

Surgical technique involves correct alignment of the two ends of the vas and the use of fine sutures to connect the two ends. Minimal tissue trauma by the surgeon is a necessity, as are the absence of bleeding, infection risk reduction by sterile fields and excellent technique. The return of sperm can be slow and semen analysis is done at between six and twelve weeks. In fact, sperm counts can continue to improve over time, even up to twelve months after the procedure. In a small percentage of men, the reversal can block off over time and they end up with no sperm again.

Successful vasectomy reversal, that is, the birth of a child, can be helped by several other factors. Having the procedure well before attempting to conceive is useful. Maximal sperm counts return slowly, so if you're aiming for conception within twelve months you might consider having the reversal now.

Also, the male should stop smoking before reversal. Microscopic blood vessels need all the help they can get to form around the reversal area, and stopping smoking will help this. I will not perform the reversal if the male is a smoker; I will only do it when they stop.

Before undergoing a vasectomy, consider the cost. It can vary and may be a significant factor for you. In Australia it is now covered by health funds and has become a lot cheaper.

Different surgeons will have different success rates, and the surgeon should have sufficient experience to offer you an excellent chance of success. Undertake thorough research.

As with all surgery, complications may occur. Obviously, the biggest complication is failure of the operation to result in an open vas deferens. Also, post-operative infection and/or a bleed or haematoma in the area are possible. My advice is to rest and lie flat for a good forty-eight hours after the operation. A TV, iPad and a couple of good books as well as an ice pack will help.

 ## Varicoceles

This term describes large varicose veins in the scrotum. The research is not conclusive as to whether varicocele repair will result in dramatic improvements in semen, however, more recent research involving the effect of this condition on sperm DNA damage is interesting.

TRAFFIC HAZARD | Freezing sperm

If you are going to have a vasectomy, consider storing some frozen sperm. There are two reasons: you and your current partner may change your mind later and want more children, or you might change partner. If you have frozen sperm, failure to reverse a vasectomy is not the end of the road. Options such as an intra-uterine insemination or even IVF are available, and you won't have to have a testicular biopsy.

Before the vasectomy you can book in at a fertility centre to freeze sperm; you will probably need a doctor's referral. You either produce a sample at home and bring it in, or produce the sample in the unit.

The sperm will be tested, and then frozen for the future. The freezing and storage costs will be advised.

I don't think permanent contraceptive methods like vasectomy are the best method any more. Socially, we are not staying in relationships like our parents did. If I see a couple who say they have finished their family and want a vasectomy or tubal ligation I try and talk them into alternative contraception, something that is easily reversible.

For example, the Mirena IUD goes into the uterus, puts out a small dose of hormone and has a contraceptive success rate equivalent to a vasectomy or tubal ligation; the statistical failure rate is approximately one in two thousand for all three. A Mirena lasts for five years, costs very little, reduces periods to little or nothing and can smooth out a female's hormonal fluctuation during her cycle.

If the couple part and a new relationship is formed and there is a desire for more children, the Mirena is simply removed and fertility is restored. It is obviously a lot simpler than a vasectomy or tubal ligation reversal.

By the way, my last two vasectomy reversals were change-of-mind couples, not new relationships.

A varicocele repair could help some men. Certainly, if the varicocele is causing pain or discomfort it requires surgery. Two methods of treatment now exist:

surgical repair, or the newer method employed by an interventional radiologist of coiling the incompetent veins higher up.

Out of position varicocele

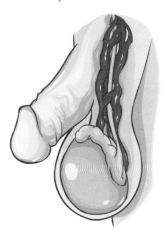

 Orchidopexy

Undescended testes in a young boy should be diagnosed early (before age one) and surgical treatment to bring the testes down and attach them in the scrotum should be performed before the age of one to two, based on current advice. This procedure is known as an orchidopexy.

Undescended testes (either unilateral or bilateral) are not uncommon in the male population. Many men are not quite sure what was done to them as a boy or if both sides were done or at what age they had it done. The later the surgery, the more risk that the sperm count will be affected significantly.

If you are affected, if possible you should ask your parents about it and get some facts. Very late orchidopexy raises the risk later in life of testicular cancer and subsequent regular ultrasounds of the testes will be required to watch for changes in the testes.

Testes in the groin or pelvis should be removed, as they pose a risk of cancer and are useless for sperm production.

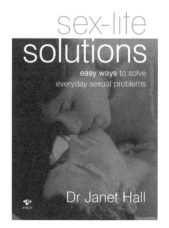

 Sex therapy

Sometimes a man may need a sex therapist to help with sex issues, an area requiring expertise as it can be quite difficult for men. Sex therapists are brilliant and have excellent success with couples that attend. They have experience in dealing with both men and women with problems like yours.

Among the patients I have referred to a therapist, the male success rates have been simply remarkable. Every successful male has made the same comment, that they wished they had been to see the therapist earlier.

The hard part, no pun intended, is that men in general do not like to talk about the problem. Sex is a topic they will rarely discuss, especially if they have a problem.

Obviously, the two big problem areas for men sexually, are impotence and libido issues. A third area would concern their partner, and it works the other way around. If you have impotence, then your partner has a sex issue as well. Always try and see it from the other point of view. A sex therapist *always* deals with couples; there may be some individual consultations, but generally they work with couples.

A brief search locally will provide you with a local specialist, although your REI infertility doctor will probably refer you to one.

ROUGH SURFACE	Summary

- Improving or fixing male fertility can be either simple or complex.
- Simple solutions include being at the right place at the right time and having more sex, changing your lifestyle and thinking about time and timing.
- Complex issues include surgery to correct vasectomies, IVF using ICSI to inject a single sperm per female egg and sex therapy.
- Male factor infertility is fixable in virtually all circumstances.
- You *can* help your own male fertility, and if not, we can help you.

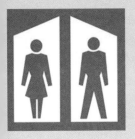

CHAPTER 14

Female infertility treatments

A s with men, the treatment options for women depend on the problem or problems.

 ## Weight

Many things affect ovulation and some problems are surprisingly simple to fix. Weight is one of these. Increases and decreases in weight can be very effective at making ovulation happen. If the patient is underweight an exercise physiologist and dietician can help them gain weight.

The target gain is 5 kg (11 lb) of fat, not muscle. Why? Because fat makes oestrogen, along with the ovaries. How many women are keen to put on 5 kg? None. However, a 5 kg weight gain will restart their reproductive hormonal system amazingly effectively. I have found this to be true over many years of practice.

For the overweight women weight loss is equally as effective. A loss of around 7 kg (15 lb) will get around 70 per cent of patients ovulating. The diets required in both circumstances are well documented and the exercise regimes are a lot simpler than people think. I suggest getting a dietician involved and taking advantage of their expertise. If weight gain or loss is suggested by your doctor or treating professional for your partner, support her by doing something practical like reducing high glycaemic index foods in the home. Also, lose some weight yourself. The best advice I can give you is: don't say too much. If your partner needs to gain weight, be supportive. If she needs to lose weight, be supportive. Don't eat take-away when she can't.

Show your support by your actions: drop the calories by dropping the beer. You don't have to say anything, as your actions will speak louder than words. And it will help if you have read something about exactly what your partner's circumstances are. If she has PCOS read up on it – knowledge will help you to understand.

Don't lecture your partner. You may be a professor of biochemistry but lecturing her will not help at all. Instead, suggest a dinner of something that is low GI. Plan meals. Make up some exercise plans and book trips to the exercise physiologist. Offer to take her. Wait there and drive her home. Be practical.

You don't need to talk too much, guys – you need to 'do'.

 Weight gain or loss will have a profound effect on fertility and on female (and male) health, as well as benefiting the foetus.

If weight is high – a BMI greater than 35, or in medical speak 'morbidly obese' – significant weight loss will be needed, to decrease the risks to the woman while pregnant. These risks include:

- gestational diabetes
- pre-eclampsia (high blood pressure and swelling)
- infection
- prolonged pregnancy (overdue)
- labour problems including anaesthetic problems
- increased risk of elective or emergency caesarean section
- increased risk of miscarriage
- increased risk of still birth
- increased risk of maternal death (rare)
- post-partum problems, including increased haemorrhage and post-natal depression

This is not a complete list, but it gives you some idea of the risks to your partner. Weight loss is also needed to decrease the risks to the foetus of:

- macrosomia, meaning a larger baby
- birth defects
- diabetes and heart disease as an adult

I have already mentioned two new areas of medicine: pre-conception medicine (before pregnancy) and peri-conception medicine (during pregnancy).

The environment before, and during, pregnancy influences the foetus and affects outcomes at birth and into the foetus' future. It took us humans a while to realise this, even though farmers had known it for ages.

Pregnancy is about two people, the mother and her child, and treating professionals have an ethical responsibility to look after both.

If you expand the thought a little it includes you. You have an awful lot invested in your partner's pregnancy – ultimately it will result in the most precious thing in your lives. You want to give these two very special people every advantage throughout the process. Reducing risks to both will provide a big advantage.

TRAFFIC HAZARD | Taking action

I once saw a couple with infertility. Both were morbidly obese: she weighed around 150 kg (330 lb) and he was closer to 180 kg (397 lb). I refused to treat them until they lost a significant amount of weight.

The man also got my lecture about being a responsible father and living until his child was old, not dying when the child was young or even having serious ill health when the child was young.

The woman cried continuously for two days. Her husband didn't. He went home and booked them in to see a surgeon who dealt in weight-loss surgery. He emptied out the pantry, larder and fridge. He organised for them to see an exercise physiologist and dietician.

Now he is almost 90 kg (198 lb) lighter and she presented to me less than one year later, nearly 50 kg (110 lb) lighter, for her first antenatal appointment. She was also beaming as she was so proud of herself and her husband.

They have three children now. No other medical treatment was ever required, just weight loss achieved by them through surgery.

'John and Jane' are my role models and mentors for any other couples I ask to lose significant weight. This lovely couple will phone others who are faced with a similar situation to tell them their story and offer support.

One last comment on weight: at a recent American Society for Reproductive Medicine conference, data was presented to show the difference in effects five years after diets as opposed to after bariatric (obesity) surgery. Diets did poorly, whereas surgery did very well. It was important to look at the five-year outcome, as short-term weight loss with diets can work but all too often fail to last.

 Weight loss surgery is highly effective. I strongly advocate this to morbidly obese patients, both male and female.

Women cannot conceive during the significant weight loss period post-surgery due to metabolic risks to the foetus, but they can as the weight loss begins to slow down.

Thyroid issues

Thyroid problems can affect ovulation and, later, the pregnancy. There are two thyroid problems: an underactive thyroid (hypothyroidism), and an overactive thyroid (hyperthyroidism).

Having an **underactive thyroid** is common. Treatment involves thyroxine daily in doses that your thyroid specialist will decide. Having an **overactive thyroid** is rare and can be managed in different ways. Most patients are given drugs to suppress the overactive thyroid, while some have treatments to permanently stop the thyroid gland and are then given thyroxine to rebalance.

Prolactin

The hormone prolactin is produced in the pituitary gland and has a role in lactation. High prolactin is generally treated with drugs; occasionally, surgery will be required. This is full-on neurosurgery but it is rare. Any prolactin-producing benign tumour in the pituitary gland must be large or not responding to medications to suppress it to warrant this.

I see high prolactin in all the literature mentioned as a cause of infertility, but professionally have rarely had to treat a case.

Ovulation induction

A series of blood tests and an occasional ultrasound scan can pinpoint ovulation. If you know exactly when your partner is ovulating, sex on that day will have the highest chance of resulting in a pregnancy.

Sometimes I need to prescribe drugs to help ovulation, and there are quite a few of these. The most common is clomiphene citrate, sold as Clomid. Clomid acts to induce ovulation by blocking oestrogen. The compensating effect is to raise oestrogen and then follicle-stimulating hormone (FSH) to induce ovulation. There are often side effects, such as headaches, nausea, visual disturbance and vaginal bleeding (called spotting). The drug can also produce mood swings.

There is a variant of clomiphene called letrozole (sold as Femara). The newer versions are aromatase inhibitors and act to block the enzyme that breaks down oestrogen. Large studies suggest they may be more effective than Clomid.

 Clomid or Femara are taken for five days from day two of the female menstrual cycle (approximately).

The specialist doctor you see will decide the drug and regime they want you to follow. Many PCOS female patients are treated with Metformin to try and reduce insulin resistance and allow things to function more normally. Hyperinsulinemia is the obvious problem, and Metformin is often the first medication written on the prescription pad. Studies show that it is less effective than clomiphene citrate or letrozole in inducing ovulation. Many endocrinologists would argue that weight loss and exercise should be the first options to treat insulin resistance as they are physiologically the better options.

If Metformin is prescribed, a simple way to start it is to build up the dose slowly to try and prevent the gastrointestinal side effects. I prescribe one tablet a day for the first week, twice a day the second week then three times a day from week three. There are obviously variations on this.

Follicle-stimulating hormone injections

Ovulation-inducing (OI) injections are synthetic FSH drugs such as Gonal-F or Puregon, which stimulate follicles to grow. The protocols for using these drugs are more involved as the risk of multiple eggs can be higher. Single-follicle ovulation is the aim.

Daily injections of an appropriate dose are given, and ultrasound scans and blood tests are used to check for follicle growth and number. The aim should be mono-follicular growth – one egg – but there can be more. Three follicles should be the maximum allowed to carry on with that cycle because of the obvious risk of twins or triplets. I cancel the cycle if there are three follicles.

TRAFFIC HAZARD	Triplets

I have had only one case where triplets were conceived (while on Clomid) from two follicles, as one egg fertilised then split into monozygotic identical twins and the other egg fertilised as a singleton. Three babies from two eggs!

Most OI protocols also involve intra-uterine insemination, so the male must produce a sample on the ovulation day. Some protocols even induce ovulation to be sure of timing and coordinate the IUI day with the laboratory – not all labs work seven days a week. Either way, men need to produce a sperm sample on the ovulation day as well as around the time of the procedure.

 ## Intra-uterine insemination

Intra-uterine insemination (IUI) is a simple technique used to create a pregnancy. With this, a male sperm is injected into the uterine cavity at the time of ovulation. This procedure is useful for men with mild sperm abnormalities. Sometimes it is used when the simple tests fail to find a cause for infertility. It is also a treatment where donor sperm can be used.

Investigations pinpoint the day of the woman's ovulation. On that day the male attends the laboratory and produces a sample of semen, which is treated to reduce it down to the best sperm. This sperm is placed in a test tube and then injected (inseminated) into the uterus.

The technique is like a simple Pap smear. A speculum is placed in the vagina, then a soft flexible catheter is inserted up through the cervix into the uterus.

The IUI technique is often associated with ovulation-inducing drugs. The ovulation-inducing drug is taken, then once ovulation is pinpointed using blood tests and perhaps also an ultrasound scan IUI is used.

 ## Surgery

There are conditions where surgery is needed to help the fertility of a woman. These conditions can be broken down into the following:

- endometriosis
- fibroids
- fallopian tubal ligation reversal

- other tubal surgery
- pelvic adhesions (scar tissues)
- uterine cavity fibroids/adhesions/congenital abnormalities or polyps

 ## Hysteroscopic surgery

This is surgery to the inside of the uterus. It is often combined with a laparoscopy, so many women undergo the combined procedure of a hysteroscopy and a laparoscopy. This will allow the surgeon to see all the reproductive anatomy.

Many reproductive specialists do a diagnostic hysteroscopy and laparoscopy first if they believe there are enough reasons in the patient's infertility history to warrant surgery. This allows a diagnosis to be followed by later operative surgery to fix the problems found.

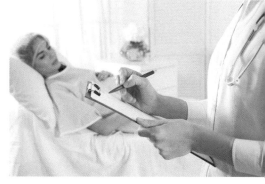

During hysteroscopic surgery the doctor will be looking for many problems, ranging from polyps, fibroids, an abnormally formed uterus shape (called congenital abnormalities) through to adhesions.

Surgery to remove polyps or simple problems may occur at the same time or later, depending on the extent of the problems found.

 ## Laparoscopic surgery

Laparoscopic, or keyhole, surgery involves two approaches. Some doctors do a diagnostic laparoscopy first to have a look and see the extent of the disease. This is a quick day surgery approach, and your partner will be in hospital for the day only. She fasts, usually from midnight, for a morning operating list, or sometimes an early breakfast is allowed for those women having an afternoon procedure. Six hours of fasting is a rough rule.

Your partner will need to be driven to the hospital and picked up, as she must not drive for twenty-four hours after an anaesthetic. Always take your partner to these procedures and pick her up. You may have a lot on in your own world, but this is very important as she is going through surgery for you both. You are there to look after her in life and this is one of those times. The surgery involves various steps. Your partner will arrive and be booked in via administration. The nurses will then admit her and check that everything is in order, check consents for the surgery, check she has been fasting and get her into a gown for surgery.

She will be nervous, so saying 'Everything will be all right' is not going to work here. Try to be supportive and acknowledge what she is going through for you both. If you think about this a bit before you get there, you will not say the wrong things. If you're unsure what to say, start simply. Ask your partner beforehand what she wants you to do on the day. Chat away about other life stuff or say little. She will give you some idea.

The anaesthetist will come in and ask a few questions. The surgeon will usually pop in for a brief chat and to ask if there are any further questions. Then your partner will be taken into theatre. Male partners leave at this point.

In theatre, she will need to get onto the operating table and a needle will be inserted into her arm. Her anaesthetist will place a mask on her to administer oxygen then will administer various drugs. One of these will put her to sleep in seconds.

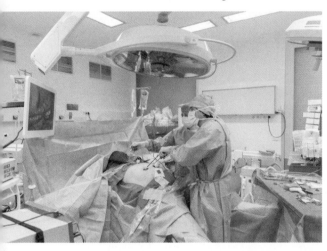

Once asleep your partner will be positioned in the lithotomy position with her legs up. Her abdomen will be swabbed with antiseptic and then special sterile drapes will be placed to cover areas not involved, exposing just the lower abdomen. If this is a diagnostic procedure most patients have a hysteroscopy first. This involves a 5 mm (0.17 in) telescope that looks in the uterine cavity, entering through the vagina and up through the cervix. Either CO_2 gas will be used to dilate the cavity and make it like a cave inside or saline fluid will more commonly be used, depending on the surgeon's preference. The telescope will be attached to a fibre optic cable and the illumination gives great views that are shown on a TV screen in the theatre. This enlarges the view greatly. The anatomy will be checked, any abnormalities noted and photos taken or sometimes a video is made. This takes less than five minutes. A special device may be left in the cervix through which to later insert dye to check the fallopian tubes. Some surgeons then proceed to surgically treat any problems they find, while some book for further surgery. It depends on the surgeon or what they find.

Next, the laparoscope will be inserted. A long, thin hollow needle (a Veress needle) will be placed through the umbilicus (belly button) and checked to confirm it is within the pelvis cavity, then CO_2 gas will be started to fill the pelvis. This is done to create a large space we can see into. CO_2 gas is used as it is safe and inert.

All of this is done to create a large safe space into which the surgeon can insert the laparoscope and other instruments. The front abdominal wall is then well away from the bowel and bladder and large blood vessels.

Other methods to create the space with CO_2 include direct entry with the 'port' or the Hasson technique, which is a small cut-down incision. Once CO_2 fills the abdomen, a larger hollow pipe (called a port) will be inserted, with a special valve on one end down which we can place instruments. The laparoscope will be attached to a camera light source then slid down the port so a view is obtained of the pelvis. A second port may be placed lower down and even more may be used, depending on the surgeon.

The pelvis will be examined systematically. The uterus will be checked, as are the ovaries and the fallopian tubes. Dye will be injected up through the cervix to check if the tubes release dye through the end. The pelvic side walls will be checked for endometriosis, adhesions (scar tissue) and fibroids and the bowel will also be reviewed. The upper abdomen will be reviewed and photos and a video taken.

If this is a diagnostic procedure it is all over. The laparoscope will be removed and the CO_2 gas released. The incisions will be sutured, and the patient will slowly wake up. The pain afterwards will be quite severe and pain relief in recovery will help this. Your partner will be ready to go home in three to four hours.

Pain will be experienced around the incision sites and, weirdly, in the shoulder due to the CO_2 gas. Rest is important. Lying flat and using good pain relief will help. It is best not to eat much afterwards, so provide small amounts of food until your partner feels hungry.

The post-operative pain from laparoscopy usually lasts a few days but can persist for up to a week in some patients. I routinely advise at least three to four days off work after it.

 ## Operative laparoscopy

Operative laparoscopy is the next step after a diagnostic, although some surgeons will go straight to this if they are sure there is endometriosis or large fibroids are present. The procedure is very similar, just longer and more complex for the surgeon.

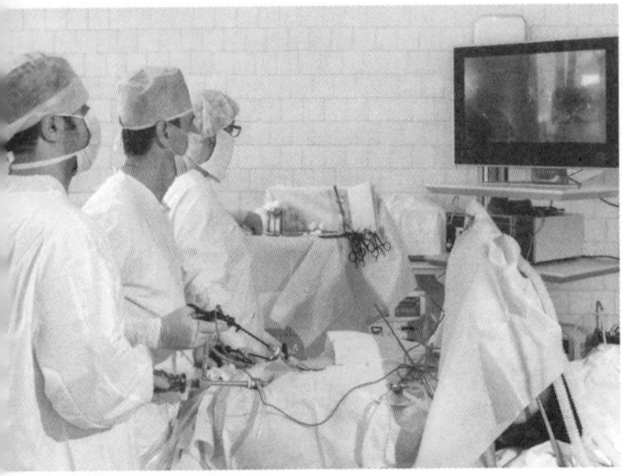

Some laparoscopic surgeons require bowel preparation beforehand to clear the bowel, as for colonoscopies. The purpose is to ensure a clean bowel in case of any bowel injury during the surgery. For one to two days before the surgery your partner will be on clear fluids and then take a preparation to clear her bowel. It's not much fun.

More complex surgery is long and painful, but recovery varies depending on the actual surgery.

Open surgery

Sometimes surgery requires an open (non-keyhole) procedure. Until the invention and then acceptance by surgeons of laparoscopic surgery, all surgery was done through a large incision. There are times where we still need to take this approach, as a fibroid may be too large or the adhesions might require open work. Sometimes complications occur during laparoscopic surgery and the patient must be opened. A major haemorrhage is one example, or perhaps a ureter injury. Recovery is longer for open operations.

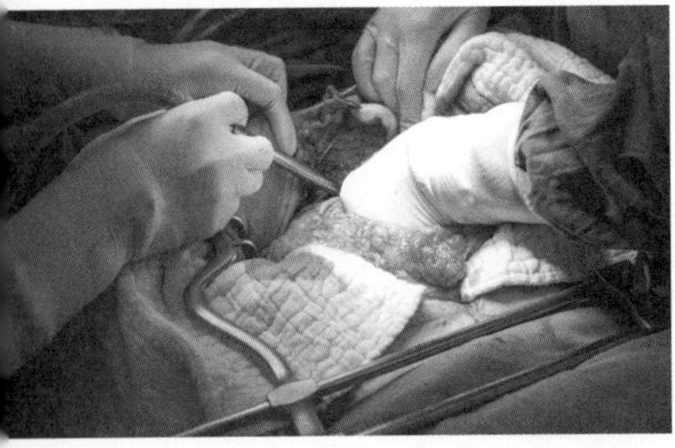

The most common incision is a horizontal one above the pubic hair line called a Pfannenstiel incision. It is about 20 cm (8 in) wide and cuts the skin, then underneath separates the two muscles called the rectus muscles. This means that no muscle is cut and recovery is better.

Occasionally, a vertical incision is required in the midline below the umbilicus. This is far more painful to recover from but gives the surgeon greater access to the abdomen if required. It's called a midline incision.

Tubal ligation reversal

Tubal ligation (sometimes called having the tubes tied) is more common than vasectomy in most countries. The procedure can be reversed.

There are two ways to do this: either through an open incision or a laparoscopic operation. Much like vasectomy reversal, it involves microsurgery – very fine sutures and a trained surgeon. The principles of repair are the same as for vasectomy repair.

Patency (open) rates for the tubes vary but pregnancy rates are around 50 to 70 per cent. You need to remember that a woman with a tubal ligation has proven fertility already, so is not necessarily the same as an infertile female. One final comment on tubal ligation reversal: at age forty-two or more it is probably a better

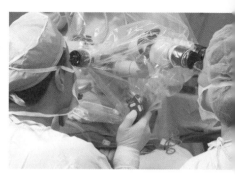

alternative than IVF. The success rates of IVF drop dramatically by that age. Tubal reversal, if successful with open tubes, gives the couple a chance at *every* ovulation, that is, approximately monthly for the next few years. Some couples are happy with that chance as they already have children (obviously) and the pressure for another is not as strong as it is for a couple with no children.

Even if the woman's chance of conceiving after surgery per month is low, say 2 to 3 per cent, when you multiply it by twelve months you get a yearly cumulative chance of 24 to 36 per cent. Those are not bad odds compared to the zero chance before the surgery.

In vitro fertilisation

In vitro fertilisation (IVF) is the most likely next procedure. It comes into its own as the only treatment if men have a low sperm count or if there are blocked tubes. Also, there are many additional reasons that IVF can be the best treatment choice. *See* Chapter 15 for more information.

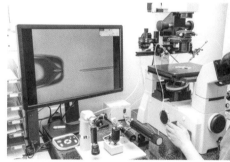

The IVF option may also depend on the doctor's practice. My approximate rate is that around 25 per cent of couples I see end up needing IVF.

IVF does exactly what its name suggests, which is 'out of the body' fertilisation. We can see this happen in the lab once the sperm and eggs are collected.

Other treatments

There are many other female treatments I have not covered in this basic chapter. For example, some Clomid patients fail to ovulate even on high doses. Medically this is called Clomid resistance, and ovarian drilling can help. Keyhole surgery is used to allow a needle to puncture the ovary multiple times, which surprisingly helps the ovary function better and ovulate. This is called laparoscopic ovarian drilling.

TRAFFIC HAZARD | Stein-Leventhal syndrome

Originally polycystic ovary syndrome was named in 1935 after two gynaecologists, Irving Stein and Michael Leventhal, who basically discovered the association of cystic ovaries and anovulation. They also operated on these ovaries and improved ovulation by cutting out a quarter of each ovary. Now we use keyhole surgery and drill (puncture) the ovary, which is just as effective and much simpler.

The use of a drug called naltrexone with Clomid-resistance can help some, although naltrexone is mainly used for opiate addiction! I believe it was discovered at drug addiction clinics that patients using it had higher pregnancy rates.

If the woman has congenital adrenal hyperplasia and makes too many male-like androgenic hormones from the adrenal gland, the use of special steroids can reduce this and allow ovulation to occur.

Sex therapy may also be required, which was discussed in Chapter 5.

Neurosurgery for a prolactinoma in the pituitary gland, raising prolactin, might be required although very rarely, as large prolactinomas (called macro prolactinomas) are rare and the drug Dostinex is very effective at reducing the prolactin level and allowing ovulation to occur.

ROUGH SURFACE | Summary

- Female treatments for infertility are designed to address the main issue of ovulation or anatomy. Ovulation is the number one problem, so it is the number one target of treatment. This can range from lifestyle changes to improve ovulation, such as weight loss or gain, simple cycle tracking to pinpoint ovulation, or the use of oral drugs like Clomid to stimulate ovulation.

- Prior to any treatment it is important to address under-lying issues such as thyroid problems. Obviously, life-style modification regarding smoking and drinking will help. Starting folate three months prior to conception is a routine practice as well.
- Surgery may help correct anatomical issues involving the fallopian tubes, endometriosis, fibroids or adhesions, by the laparoscopic or open approach.
- In some circumstances IVF can be the best alternative.
- There are many other possible treatment options the doctors may use, depending on the female cause of infertility.

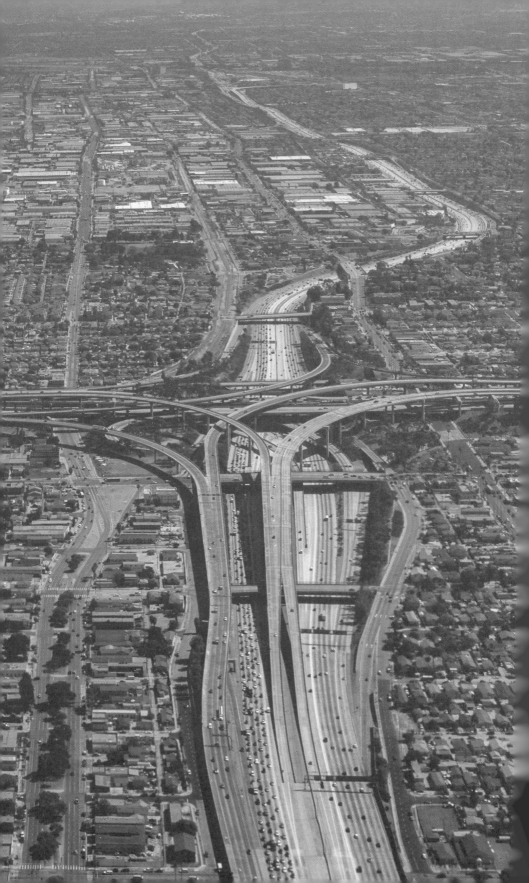

CHAPTER 15

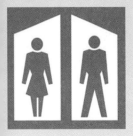

In vitro fertilisation

In vitro fertilisation (IVF) has become a common treatment for infertile couples since the first IVF baby, Louise Brown, was born in 1978, and is particularly useful for male factor problems, even though assisting men was not its original intent. Injecting a single sperm per egg (ICSI) arrived on the IVF scene about 1991.

IN VITRO FERTILISATION

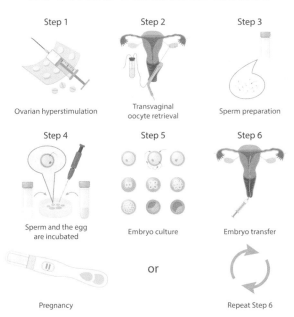

Step 1 — Ovarian hyperstimulation

Step 2 — Transvaginal oocyte retrieval

Step 3 — Sperm preparation

Step 4 — Sperm and the egg are incubated

Step 5 — Embryo culture

Step 6 — Embryo transfer

or

Pregnancy

Repeat Step 6

In vitro (*outside the body*) as compared to in vivo (*inside the body*) is the process of collecting eggs and sperm separately, fertilising them in a laboratory dish and then replacing them in the female uterus as an embryo. This is clever. The understanding and technology that allows us to see such reproductive biology at work has opened a route to fertility that never existed before. It's still a very new science in the scheme of things if you consider the span of human history.

It might not have been the route you intended to take but it may prove to be the best way to get where you want to go. More than seven million babies have been born since this method was discovered by Dr Patrick Steptoe, a UK-based gynaecologist, who conceived the idea of IVF and recruited Dr Robert Edwards,

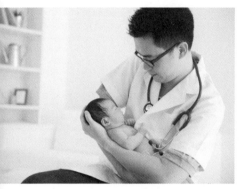

an animal reproductive scientist, to help him in 1963. He was trying to work out how to overcome tubal-factor infertility, or blocked fallopian tubes. Somehow, he had to join the egg and sperm together outside the body.

In 1977 they succeeded, and Louise Brown was born on 25 July 1978.

Her birth was the result of a single egg collected laparoscopically by Steptoe. No drugs were used in her IVF, which was a 'natural' cycle. Drug treatments to stimulate more eggs had not then been developed. IVF has two advantages – its strongest features! We see the sperm fertilise the egg and the embryo returned to its natural environment. Its advantage is captured in the name.

The second advantage is unique to this form of assisted reproductive technology (ART). Embryos can be frozen if there are extra embryos after the first transfer of an embryo. If desired, during that first cycle all embryos can be frozen for future use.

 IVF has two main advantages. First, you see the egg and sperm fertilise and make an embryo. Second, you can freeze embryos.

That is a huge advantage. A frozen embryo cycle is simple: it is relatively inexpensive, and my particularly favourite aspect is that it *preserves* the fertility potential of that embryo at the age of the woman when it was made in the lab. If she was thirty-two, the embryo has a thirty-two-year-old's potential to implant and make a baby; if she was twenty-eight, a twenty-eight-year-old's and so on. Frozen embryos do not age at all. They do not degenerate, and my reading suggests that if stored properly in liquid nitrogen at –196°C (–320°F), they could last as long as fifty thousand years before cosmic radiation damaged them. With new freezing techniques called vitrification, freezing is now quite straightforward.

When IVF is the best choice

If a man has a very low sperm count, or very slow sperm, then natural fertility is virtually impossible. For men with these problems IVF is the only option to achieve a pregnancy using the couple's sperm and eggs.

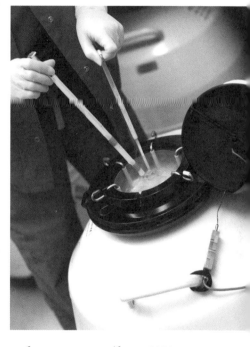

Early IVF couldn't help men with low sperm numbers, poor motility, even significant shape abnormalities; they had poor IVF success rates. The eggs and sperm were collected and then placed in a petri dish to fertilise.

Then, a single IVF egg was placed in a special dish with a specific number of sperm – 50,000 to 150,000 sperm per egg depending on sperm quality. By the following morning fertilisation should have occurred in most eggs, but poor sperm equalled poor fertilisation and for thirteen to fourteen years (from 1978 to 1991) results were always the same. If the male's sperm was of poor quality, then fertilisation rates were terrible. Men were advised to get a sperm donor.

Intracytoplasmic sperm injection: the wonder injection

A useful discovery occurred by accident. It was believed that injecting a single sperm into an egg was unsafe. Scientists used to try to slip a sperm beneath the shell of the egg, called the zona, but outside the cytoplasm. Think of it as being placed under the shell of a hen's egg (except the human shell is much softer), but outside the white.

Dr Gianpiero Palermo, at a Belgium IVF unit in Brussels, injected a sperm directly into the cytoplasm by accident. When he realised his mistake, he

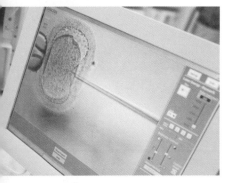

planned to discard the egg but then decided to leave it until morning to see what happened. The following morning, he found that the egg had been fertilised. It progressed to an embryo.

Sperm injection techniques, known as intracytoplasmic sperm injections (ICSI) changed the face of IVF. Nowadays the technique is used in approximately 50 per cent of all IVF uses to improve fertilisation rates.

 Protocols

There are several IVF protocols to stimulate the female to grow eggs:

- Natural IVF: no drugs are used, and a single egg is collected. This is rarely used now.
- Clomid stimulation: higher doses can stimulate more eggs to grow than would naturally. One of the early IVF protocols was developed in Australia; it produced more eggs than natural ovulation. Now it is rarely used.
- Long down regulation IVF: drugs turn off the female's hormones, keep them turned off, then synthetic FSH drugs stimulate the ovaries to grow eggs.
- Short cycle IVF: synthetic FSH drugs start to grow eggs, and then another drug is added to stop sudden ovulation.
- Short cycle IVF with long-acting FSH drugs: this is like the protocol above but with fewer injections.
- Flare cycles: most suppressing hormones work by turning on (agonist) the hormone they will ultimately suppress. The initial days it 'flares' FSH. We can use this effect.

Over the years doctors have come up with many unique ways to stimulate egg growth.

TRAFFIC HAZARD	Hormones

- GnRH is made in the hypothalamus and then acts on the pituitary gland to release FSH and LH.
- The synthetic drug given to block GnRH (for example, Lucrin injection or Syneral nasal spray) is known as a GnRH agonist. It works by initially stimulating GnRH (a flare)

but then depletes the hypothalamic stores of GnRH and effectively blocks it. It is given daily during the IVF cycle.

- Another synthetic drug to block GnRH is known as a GnRH antagonist. It works directly by blocking GnRH with no flare (for example, Orgalutran).
- FSH is made in the pituitary and then acts via the blood stream on the ovary, to grow a follicle (the small 2 cm fluid-filled sac with an egg inside).
- Synthetic FSH is used as a daily injection to stimulate the ovary to grow follicles (for example, Puregon or Gonal-F).
- LH is made in the pituitary and then acts via the blood stream on the ovary, to cause ovulation, the act of the egg being released from the follicle.
- Synthetic LH is occasionally given to assist follicle development (for example, Luveris).
- Some hormone injections combine FSH and HVG (for example, Menopur).
- HCG acts like LH but for much longer. It is called the 'trigger' injection to stimulate ovulation. This is sometimes given after embryo transfer during the luteal phase (for example, Pregnyl or Ovidrel).
- Progesterone is given after embryo transfer to support the luteal phase (for example, Crinone).

Let's walk through a basic agonist and the antagonist protocol, probably the two most common IVF protocols in the world.

Each IVF unit will have variations on this so just use this as a guide, not a rule book.

Step 1   The reproductive doctor recommends IVF for a good reason – let's make this a male-factor issue with a low, slow semen analysis. The test has been repeated twice and there has been no change.

Step 2   Referral to the IVF unit and a nurse interview. The procedure and steps are explained to the couple. The nurse shows both partners how to use the needles, sets doses, and outlines many more practical parts of the process. They will also discuss consents for the IVF that each unit has individually produced. The financial costs are consented to and this is finalised.

Step 3   The protocol is outlined, and drug prescriptions or actual drugs given to the couple. The first drug is called a GnRH agonist. Agonists stimulate GnRH in the hypothalamus initially but then deplete the stores of GnRH and effectively act to suppress it. Suppressing GnRH suppresses production by the pituitary gland of FSH and LH, chemically shutting down the female reproductive hormones. This is like menopause: if you cut the fuel line to a car motor the engine will shut down. Its main effect is to prevent a sudden rise in natural LH, which would cause each follicle to ovulate the egg. Natural (that is, the female's own) LH is triggered by the rising oestrogen, so stopping this happening is vital so that eggs are there when we do an egg collection. Commonly this drug is administered by daily injections or by daily nasal spray.

Step 4   The blood tests and ultrasound scan start to check hormone levels and ovaries.

Step 5   Once the female hormones are suppressed by the GnRH agonist, synthetic FSH is started; there are two daily injections. This stimulates follicles to grow and, hopefully, within each follicle a small egg is growing. Commonly, it may take ten to twelve days to grow a batch of eggs but the range can be from eight to eighteen days.

TRAFFIC HAZARD | The jab man

Did I mention that often you men have to give these injections? You need to help here. The IVF nurses will teach you, and your partner will appreciate it.

You might think of trying to get out of it because you:

- don't like needles and they turn you into a wimp
- are terrified of hurting your partner
- don't want to have anything to do with the whole thing
- are legally blind
- worry she will hate you for doing the injecting (she won't, or else she must do the injecting)
- have no arms (not the same as being harmless)

I have news for you: you are going to do it because it is the right thing to do. You are not on the sharp end of the needle or getting the hormones. Become the best injecting partner on the planet – and do it with a laugh and a sense of humour.

Step 6 (a) The trigger injection. When enough eggs have grown for long enough the doctor will decide your partner is ready for a trigger. A trigger stimulates ovulation and is analogous to the LH rise, which is what naturally stimulates the egg to be released, ready to meet a sperm, and to switch on meiosis (halves the chromosomes from forty-six to twenty-three per egg).

We use a drug like LH that is longer acting, because we have suppressed the patient's hormones and the longer-acting LH (called HCG) supports the woman's endometrium, ready for embryo transfer five days after the egg pick up. Most injections to trigger are given the evening two days before egg collection. It's an exact number of hours to allow the unit to schedule the IVF egg collection. Pioneering IVF could not control the LH rise so egg collections happened at any hour, including nights. Thankfully, that problem has been solved.

For instance, if your partner is booked for her egg collection at 10 am on Wednesday the trigger will be given at 10 pm the Monday before. This also allows us a window of time to do the egg collection before the egg ovulates. Usually it is about four hours. Lists can be rearranged; issues can arise and so forth.

Step 6 (b) Trigger with the agonist. Occasionally we decide that for several reasons we will trigger with the agonist and not the HCG. This can only be during an antagonist cycle. Simply put, the agonist blocks the antagonist, allowing the patient's natural LH to surge and cause ovulation. It may be used if the woman has too many eggs growing, and we are concerned about ovarian hyper-stimulation syndrome (OHSS). With this unique condition, the IVF sometimes causes blood vessels to leak fluids; if severe, it may require hospitalisation. In this case we still do an egg collection but don't do an embryo transfer. This is called a freeze all (embryos) cycle.

Step 7   Egg collection. This is scheduled precisely: the egg is naturally released approximately thirty-six hours after the start of the LH surge or twelve hours after the LH peak. We simulate this with our synthetic LH equivalent but do the egg pick-up a bit earlier. That way they are still in the follicle, switched on (they have halved their chromosomes ready to meet a sperm with its half chromosomes), and the timing suits the IVF unit for egg collection. We try to do this in the mornings so that busy IVF scientists can work with the eggs and sperm in office hours.

There are different ways of doing an egg collection, depending on whether this is a standard stimulation IVF cycle aiming for ten to fourteen eggs or a low stimulation protocol IVF cycle aiming for three to six eggs.

Standard protocol IVF egg collection

Egg collection is either done in an operating theatre or a special room in the clinic. A minor anaesthetic is given to the woman, either by the IVF doctor or an anaesthetist. Some units may just give light sedation – it can vary. A transvaginal scan is done to check the ovaries and follicles. Local anaesthetic may be injected to numb the vagina. A special IVF needle is attached to the transvaginal probe.

When the doctor is happy with their view, they advance the needle into the ovary and into the first follicle. A small suction pump on the needle sucks the follicular fluid out and into a test tube. The test tube is passed to a waiting scientist with a microscope and they search for an egg. If an egg is found, the doctor then moves the needle into another follicle and so on. Both ovaries are drained of all possible eggs. Only the larger follicles have eggs, and all are drained.

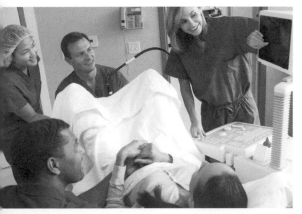

Most units show the eggs to the couple each time one is found. The whole procedure generally takes less than thirty minutes. Total egg numbers vary considerably from patient to patient depending on multiple factors such as age, if they have PCOS, response of the ovary to that IVF cycle, drug dose and so on. The average is around ten to twelve eggs per egg collection.

TRAFFIC HAZARD | Low-cost protocol IVF egg collection

In this case the egg collection may not require a theatre but just a procedure room to avoid hospital costs. Pre-medication such as Valium and Panadol with codeine is given approximately one hour before. The actual collection is done with a gas such as nitrous oxide (laughing gas). Local anaesthetic may or may not be used.

These collections may have fewer eggs (some have the normal egg numbers) to collect and are typically quick – six to seven minutes in total. That's my average.

If you see the needle used for the egg collection, please try not to faint. It is approximately 35 cm (14 in) long and the biggest needle you will ever behold. I try to not let the woman see it until we have finished the procedure.

Some men see it, go white and look very worried. It's important not to falter; stay the course and look after your partner. And remember, it's not you that the needle is pointing at. Some units don't allow the male partner to be present at the egg collection procedure.

Step 8   The male finally has his job to do – a semen collection is required. The routine is the same as for previous semen collections. All those 'years of training as a teenager', as one male patient informed me, are finally put to some good use. Men who are very nervous can have a previous sample frozen as a back-up.

Step 9   Your partner goes to recovery for an hour or so and then home to rest. She should rest up for the day and lie flat. The male should look after her and not claim he needs to recover too and he should not go back to work that day! Look after her. It hurts having your eggs sucked out, as I am frequently reminded by patients.

Plan to give your partner regular Panadol, hot packs, a nice place for her to rest and a few good books or magazines to read. Maybe you could organise a DVD or Netflix to watch. If you went through a procedure (and some will to have sperm surgically removed) you would expect no less.

Step 10   The scientists in the laboratory get to work on the sperm and eggs. The decision whether to do IVF and inseminate a single egg with many thousands of sperm is usually already made. In some cases, they will do ICSI and inject a single sperm into a single egg. How?

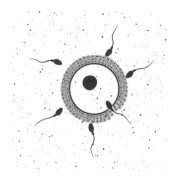

The eggs are placed in a special fluid, then they are stripped of their surrounding cumulus cells until just the egg is seen.

Using microsurgical equipment, the egg is locked in place. The sperm have been treated and the best ones selected to be used. They are wiggly, motile sperm like fast-moving tadpoles. Various techniques have been used to slow them down to a speed that the scientist can deal with. One involves a light blow to the head: seriously! It literally stuns the sperm enough for the scientist to suck it into a small syringe. Then the sperm is injected into the cytoplasm (white) of the egg. The eggs have been deemed mature after a thorough microscopic review. Every mature egg is injected with a good single sperm. It is time consuming, particularly if a lot of eggs were collected.

Step 11 For the man and woman not much happens at this point. Some female blood tests are needed. If she is well, plans are set in place for the embryo transfer.

A cycle is divided into two parts. The first part is growing eggs – called the follicular part. Follicles are those small fluid-filled sacs I described earlier. Inside each, hopefully, is a tiny little egg. We just went and got them. The phase after is called the luteal phase, named after the corpus luteum. If you recall, an egg grows in the follicle then ovulates out or is collected by IVF. The follicle remains, now called the corpus luteum, and starts to produce progesterone (in the natural situation, but not during IVF). It is waiting to sense the embryonic hormone HCG and, if it does, make huge doses of progesterone to support the early pregnancy. We need to support the IVF luteal phase with either progesterone (which the patient can't naturally make due to drugs) or small doses of the HCG. HCG was used for the trigger in a big dose. Your own IVF unit should explain the process, but feel free to ask. You need to understand IVF, and the better you do the more it helps you and your partner.

Step 12 On day three or five after the egg collection, depending on the IVF unit, an embryo will be selected by the scientist for transfer. When the couple arrives, some bureaucratic paperwork will be completed. The scientist usually has a chat to them about the embryos they have available. This may range from just one through to many, but an average might be one to three. The discussion will include quantity and quality of the embryos. They are shown the embryos on a TV screen in the theatre.

The transfer is usually simple. The principle is to place the embryo within a syringe attached to a fine catheter, which is then inserted through the cervix into the uterine cavity. Some doctors use ultrasound to help them position the placement of the embryo, some don't. Simple transfers take a few minutes; harder ones can take a long time.

TRAFFIC HAZARD — Transfer numbers

The number of embryos for actual transfer is important. One is best, and we call this single embryo transfer SET. Modern freezing techniques are so good that freezing any other extra embryos is possible. A singleton pregnancy with one baby is the safest.

One embryo is best in most circumstances. I often hear: 'Just put two back, Doc, and get it over with' from patients. But rearing twins is not easy. Ask anyone if having two kids at the same time is easy.

Medically, twins carry more risks.

Single embryo transfer during IVF is very much the Australian way, and we are strong advocates for this.

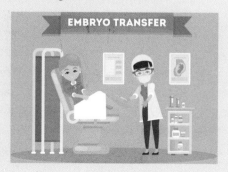

EMBRYO TRANSFER

Step 13   After the transfer the couple leaves the IVF unit. Various advice will be offered and some women are given what's called luteal (post-ovulation) support – either through injections or with tablets to place in the vagina.

My advice is to head off and have something to eat with lots of chocolate. Chocolate has serotonin in it, a 'feel good' chemical.

I advise sex for the next few nights. I politely add the word 'gentle' sex at this point. The seminal fluid acts on the endometrium to activate a whole lot of useful genes. These genes then cause the release of chemicals such as growth factors to help implantation.

Finally, I advise comedy. Yes! Laugh a lot for the next few days. An Israeli study of two hundred and twenty-nine women undergoing IVF showed an improvement in results with this approach. Google 'clown and IVF' – they used a medical 'clown'. The old saying 'laughter is the best medicine' is true.

Step 14   Wait eleven to thirteen days for the blood test to see if a positive HCG result is returned.

Practically all my patients tell me this is the hardest part. Up until then, it's all appointments, drugs, the procedure and talks to nurses, the doctor and scientists. Then … waiting.

What is your part in all this? Obviously, you are 50 per cent of the genetic DNA provided as a sperm sample, a vital role, but you have a lot more to do. You should thoroughly understand the steps in the IVF process. You should have carefully read the consents through. You should make sure the financial side is sorted out.

But the best thing you can do is communicate with your partner: talk about the IVF process. There are the factual parts to consider. Have a good feel for what is happening and when, why it is happening and what the next step will be. There are also emotional parts. It's emotionally challenging, so talk about that. Random chats can be good; arranged chats can be better. I advise making a time each day to talk about IVF before it starts and during – perhaps for thirty minutes after the main course at dinner. A pen and paper to scribble on helps identify areas of concern and provides a focus.

You're both going through IVF; you're both stressed about it, so supporting each other is good. It's well worth getting some extra support; an outside person to speak with can really help and you should suggest and support this. A mum, sister, friend or colleague can be very helpful for your partner. Sometimes you will need someone to chat to about it. Try and find a good supportive listener rather than someone who gives advice too readily.

I saw a couple recently who have done many cycles and the male had never talked to a friend about it – not even once. Try it; it helps.

 ## Aspects to consider

There are many aspects to IVF. Here are a few well worth remembering:

- It is a process of *probabilities*: a younger woman has a higher probability of a pregnancy per chance than an older woman.
- If a woman is older she has less chance per go, but don't give up after just one or two tries.
- IVF costs money: this varies around the world, from zero cost in some countries that cover IVF through to tens of thousands per try in countries that have no governmental support. Do your research on costs and check the IVF unit's pregnancy rates. This is vital.
- Don't panic about costs: by definition, infertility means that your partner is not pregnant and probably is still in the workforce earning income. If she was on maternity leave or back at work with childcare or a nanny, the costs of being off work or supporting the child are high. Financially, infertile couples are well ahead. A lawyer in Sydney once complained to me about IVF costs. My brief, back-of-the-envelope financial assessment of her financial gain over four years of infertility, making senior partner at the legal practice, not working part time, not having nannies and so forth was enormous: well over a million dollars. I pointed this out to her and she reluctantly acknowledged that my maths was sound. I know it's not fair that you and your partner need IVF and her annoying friends are all having sex and conceiving easily, but this is how the cards have been dealt.
- Sort out your lifestyle well before undergoing IVF. Don't smoke, don't drink, and start the pre-pregnancy multivitamins as recommended by your GP. Update any vaccinations as required.
- Understand the IVF process well. I know I have said this before, but it bears repeating.
- You don't need to know all about the drugs we use (but we can tell you lots if you want). You do need to know where appointments are and when. You need to know what to have read before you arrive, what to bring, what to wear, when to fast before a procedure. You need to know how many days of abstinence are required before a sample of sperm

is given. You should know your medical insurance details. Check if you're covered for IVF; if not, maybe upgrade. Upgrade to include obstetrics also! You must have a positive attitude to IVF that it will work and one day soon a pregnancy will be happening. Sort out any leave from work that's necessary. Break it down into small parts. Start with yourself, then think about your partner. Write stuff down. Ask questions if you're unsure, either by phone or email to the IVF unit.

- Be patient: you can be positive, but you don't know how it's all going to go. Will it work this time? It's emotionally challenging, so try to not be overwhelmed. Maybe fewer eggs are made than you expected. Maybe the cycle is cancelled because of overstimulation (too many eggs) or too few eggs. Remain solid.
- IVF is a lot like cooking – getting the recipe right is vital. Most of the time an IVF cycle goes well, but sometimes the doctors need to change the recipe. Each couple is different and has unique issues.
- IVF keeps getting better – the process is always being refined and improved – but, ultimately, it depends on the quality of the eggs and sperm.
- Trust your doctor and their IVF team. If you have done your research and have a good unit, they want this to work as much as you do. IVF units are judged by what is called the 'take home baby' rate. It's what we do to make babies!
- IVF really is Mother Nature at work (with some human manipulation). It's an amazingly complex process where a sperm and an egg get together to form another human. We physically help it happen, but the process is inbuilt into each sperm and each egg.

Pre-cancer treatment IVF

Several times a year I get a call from an oncologist to urgently see a couple where one of the partners has been found to have cancer. We can do an IVF cycle quickly to collect eggs from the female, make embryos then freeze them. Chemotherapy may damage the ovarian egg stores, and this is a reproductive insurance technique. Single females can do IVF and freeze eggs only. Males can freeze sperm but that does not require IVF, just a semen sample collected then frozen. This may sound easy, but many men diagnosed with cancer are very sick and producing a sample by masturbation can be virtually impossible. We can do a quick testicular biopsy in those circumstances.

I was recently asked to get sperm from a young, terribly ill man with leukaemia. The trouble was he was one of the sickest patients I have ever seen. Masturbation to produce a sample was like climbing Mount Everest to him. I couldn't biopsy him for medical reasons to do with potentially allowing leukaemic cells into his testes. After discussions with the oncologist we delayed chemo for two days, used a special filter to get white blood cells (the leukaemic) out of his blood, then gave him Viagra. Amazingly, he produced a sample on each day. We froze the second days' sample, then he started chemo. 'Hey doc! I come in here for cancer and I get asked to empty my pipes!' he joked. It was an incredible case.

 ## Donor IVF

IVF can can donor operation donor egg. The alternation for the former is where the male partner has no sperm. The process of IVF is the same, except donor sperm is used. Before that point a lot has happened and there are counselling and legal aspects to be worked through, but the process in the lab is the same.

Similarly, IVF can be used with donor eggs. The female egg donor goes through the IVF process – once again after a lot of counselling, legal processes and so on. The made embryo is transferred back into the female partner, not the donor. This can take a bit of co-ordinating to get the two women synchronous, but we are good at this. Donor egg cycles are used for egg issues and particularly where female age has become a huge problem. You can be almost certain any IVF pregnancy related in the media for a woman aged forty-five or over is from an egg donor cycle. Very few ever acknowledge this.

 ## Egg freezing

IVF can be used for egg freezing, where the woman goes through IVF and the collected eggs are frozen for the future. You may have seen this in the news. Companies like Google and Facebook are offering it to their female employees! I recently set this up for a female relative who found out she had cancer at the age of eighteen. I couldn't do much about the cancer, but two minutes after finding out I called a colleague in her city and set up an urgent IVF cycle to get her to produce eggs and freeze them before the chemotherapy started. The oncologist and fertility specialist had a great working relationship and co-ordinated it perfectly.

Egg freezing can also be used for social reasons. For example, a female patient flew in from Europe to do an IVF cycle to freeze her eggs as insurance against the future. She has a remarkable position in her profession in Europe and the

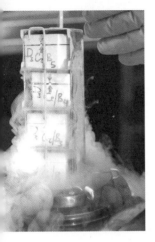

trajectory she is on means she doesn't feel she can stop to have children until around age forty-five. At thirty she froze her eggs for use in the future. It is not guaranteed that they will work, or that she will have enough frozen. You need a decent number to have any hope – at least six but probably ten to twelve is better and some recent studies suggest twenty. The new technique of vitrification, snap freezing, is much better than were previous techniques. After drawing the fluid out of the egg by osmosis using special sugary fluids, the egg, which looks like a dried raisin, is snap frozen in liquid nitrogen at −196°C (−320°F). It can remain frozen safely virtually forever.

Pre-implantation genetic diagnosis

The embryo created by IVF can also in some cases be genetically tested. This is done if either there is a known genetic condition in the mother or father or simply to look for genetic problems, and is known as pre-implantation genetic diagnosis (PGD).

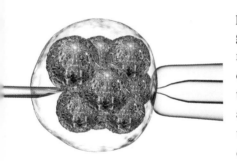

PGD might be used if for example the parents had a previous child with a severe genetic condition, for example, Duchenne muscular dystrophy, a complex muscular disease. The gene is identified in the parent, then embryos can be tested, and the non-affected embryo transferred back into the uterus. Testing is done by removing a few cells from the embryo and sending them off for testing. Usually the embryo is then frozen until the result of testing is complete. Common genetic condition examples include cystic fibrosis, fragile X, thalassemia, Tay-Sachs disease and haemophilia.

PGD can also select for diseases that only affect males, for example, sex-linked diseases. The mutation is carried on the X chromosome, but because males do not have a normal X chromosome to balance the abnormal one they are affected. The women with one abnormal gene and one normal are called carriers. Even if the gene cannot be identified the male embryo can be, and is not transferred. Haemophilia and Duchenne's are examples of X-linked diseases.

PGD can also help for gene faults that may potentially affect the embryo in later years, for example, the cancer gene BRCA1. Testing for this gene in an embryo then not transferring those embryos effectively removes that gene from the gene pool, and it can no longer affect the family and generations to follow.

PGS involves screening the embryos for genetic mistakes and is often used throughout the world. Normal (euploid) embryos can then be transferred back. Nature makes many abnormal embryos and PGS reduces the time to pregnancy by not using these abnormal (aneuploid) embryos.

PGD may be combined with PGS. The mutated gene is identified in the embryo, which is also screened for other genetic mistakes. Sometimes the embryo without the disease gene is abnormal in other ways, and vice versa. It is a large topic, so I won't go into it here.

Surrogacy

Surrogacy is where the made embryo is transferred back to another female to carry the pregnancy; it can only be achieved by the IVF process. The surrogate carries the foetus for nine months and delivers it, and the couple who made the embryo become the parents they dreamed of being. This solution is for a woman who lacks a uterus or is not allowed to carry a pregnancy for medical reasons.

Surrogacy is medically complicated and legally quite involved. It can take up to a year to get fully organised with medical opinions, legal, psychiatric and psychological issues. This is all done so that moving forward the commissioning couple and the surrogate are fully informed, psychologically assessed to handle the burden it places, and covered legally. To carry someone else's baby for nine months then give it back is quite an ask, and must be set up and managed well. Our surrogacy cases go to an independent board for final approval.

Some people may say surrogacy is wrong, but I don't agree. It is ethically and morally justifiable and acceptable. One of the reasons I did a Masters in Bioethics was to understand the ethical side of reproductive medicine. Genetically the embryo and baby are from a couple's own sperm and eggs. A 'host' carries the pregnancy and returns it after providing the incubator for nine months. Without doubt this is one of the greatest gifts ever. In some ways it is simpler than using a donor egg or donor sperm, as the embryo is yours genetically and returns to you as your child. The surrogate can either do this out of the goodness of their heart, or for commercial reasons. Right now, commercial surrogacy is illegal in Australia, but it is being reviewed.

ROUGH SURFACE	Summary

- IVF is the most involved of all infertility treatments. For some couples, it is the only possible treatment if the fallopian tubes are blocked or the semen analysis shows low parameters for the male. But there are many other circumstances where it is a very good thing, including if there has been a diagnosis of cancer
- Many couples will travel this road if they have infertility. Developing a thorough understanding of the process is like reading up on your route before leaving: once the journey has started, you will recognise the features along the way.
- IVF is an amazing fertility road trip.
- If it's your path, good luck!

CHAPTER 16

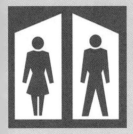

Further options: the roads less travelled

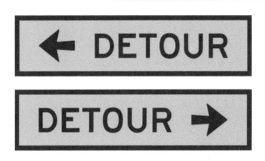

There are many and varied treatments for infertility but sometimes no matter what we try they do not work. In that case other options to meet the desire for parenthood must be considered.

I have found that many couples consist of different personalities working together. I call it the yin and yang effect – opposites attract. She may be an organiser-perfectionist, he is the laid-back type; there are many versions. This makes for a good mix of personalities. She loves his relaxed attitude and he her organisation, and in good times it works well.

Infertility, like most illnesses, exaggerates the differences and that can be difficult. She wants to know everything about it, researches, obsesses and broods. Her multi-tasking brain keeps thinking about it all the time. He, on the other hand, takes his usual approach of 'what will be, will be' and worries only a little or ignores it. His total-tasking brain puts it aside and deals only with other issues in life. Conflicts may arise because they approach the infertility problem differently. Yet, underneath this they both want the same thing: a child or children. The differences are a good thing! Be aware of them and use them. Too many couples find the differences confusing and upsetting and the cause of more conflict.

Who teaches a couple how to deal with major issues like infertility or even their own differences? Most parents don't. Schools don't. There are hundreds of books that do cover infertility, but men rarely read them. Men should understand that if an issue is emotional it is probably important.

Infertility is not a new thing; it has been part of the human experience since humans began. It was a common part of human existence and initially there were no treatments. The advent of IVF sometimes lulls couples into a false confidence that they are guaranteed a baby if they just try hard enough. Sadly, that is not the case and it can be a devastating discovery. But it is not the end of the road.

'Failed' fertility treatments

Some couples must face failed fertility treatment after having long ago entered the world of infertility. It might be the result of multiple failed IVF cycles, and

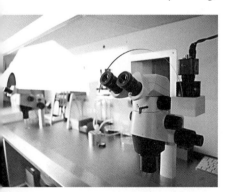

doctors have advised them to consider not going further, given the failure.

It has such a final ring to it doesn't it? *Failed.* You've tried, and you have failed. Like an exam in life, you didn't pass. That's how many people, and particularly men, feel about it. The male partner is supposed to fix things, not fail.

As hard as it is, you must believe the truth: you *did not* fail. It's simply not that kind of situation. You did everything you possibly could; as the saying goes: 'Life is like a game of cards – you can only play with the hand you are dealt.'

But how do you move on?

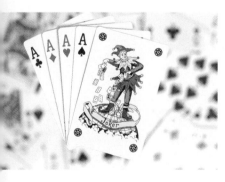

Get a second opinion

For some people the best option is to get a second or even a third opinion from another reproductive medicine doctor. That doctor can get all the available information to date and review it thoroughly with hindsight. Some units run clinics for recurrent IVF failure. The tests that are then undertaken search out the rare causes, the minutiae at the edges.

I once saw a lovely couple who had had a late miscarriage after a long period of infertility. I was that second opinion. I diligently took a full history from both. At some point I talked to them about common causes presenting commonly, common causes presenting uncommonly and uncommon causes presenting rarely. This is like saying that Fords and Toyotas present commonly, sometimes uncommonly, and Ferraris are rare.

Years later, as this couple's situation became more and more complicated, the woman started to refer to herself as the 'pink Ferrari'. She had a rare uterine anomaly – approximately a quarter of her uterus didn't develop properly. She found the only research paper on this matter in a French medical journal and had it translated for me. The male partner had a rare chromosomal problem – his sperm had the wrong number of chromosomes. We ended up using donor sperm and they now have two children.

My favourite new parents, Gary and Sue, had previously undergone *thirty-two* failed IVF cycles. I was their third or fourth opinion during ten years of trying. They now have two children.

The statistical pregnancy rate for a couple per IVF cycle is unknown. We can only work with larger statistics that reflect age, causes of infertility and the quality and quantity of embryos.

It is well worth a second opinion. You may have to do your own research in your area to decide who to see. You might consider travelling to another city for a review by a doctor and their team there. It's like finding a good tradesman in your home town: you rely on word of mouth and an endorsement from someone else. Doctors are no different, so do some digging.

TRAFFIC HAZARD	How many children do you want?

When I see a couple, I ask how many children they wanted before infertility became an issue. The usual answer is 'just one'. Often, that means they are desperate for 'just one'. I ask how many children they wanted once upon a time and they usually say two to three. I tell them my aim is to give them the number of children they first desired, the number they might have had if there were no problems, and I work towards this. It influences how I treat each couple. It's a big question and a good question. Infertility, in a way, is another

(Cont.)

illness and doctors try to return patients to the status quo: reduce blood pressure, treat cholesterol, prevent and treat asthma to allow a normal life and normal life expectancy. This is a good aim.

How you achieve children might not be how you imagined once early on in your relationship. IVF might be required, donor sperm or eggs, adoption even surrogacy. But try for the family you once envisioned.

Knowing when to stop

Having said all that, how will you know when you've reached the point where

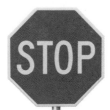

you want to stop? Are you allowing yourselves a set number of IVF tries before you stop? How would you determine what the correct number is? Have you and your partner discussed this recently?

You need to have a plan.

Life can be approached on multiple levels: intellectually (*mind*), emotionally (*heart*), spiritually (*soul*), and with persistence (*strength*).

If you focus on an intellectual approach you will miss the emotional component. Think too emotionally and you miss the intellectual side. The soul side of things is about what you may or may not believe; spiritual belief can help some people through the infertility situation.

You will need to maintain your strength to get through this trial. You may be strong, or your partner may be, or perhaps you both are. Sometimes you both lose strength and must get it from others.

Communication

Communication is often not a strong point for men, who are more inclined to action. As author John Gray says in *Men Are from Mars, Women Are from Venus*, men fix problems. Infertility problems are issues we might not be able to fix. Talking about this might be hard, but we should make the effort. The question is how to best do it.

When I ask a couple into my room for a consult on infertility, be it in Australia, Ireland, New Zealand or England, I notice the same behaviours. Women look up and smile and men rarely do. My rough approximation would be that greater than 90 per cent of women smile and fewer than 2 per cent of men do. This seems to me to be basic human behaviour.

Seeing a doctor is stressful. Men do what they do in times of stress and act like their forefathers did – then suppress emotion. Women are obviously more emotional and certainly more readable. They are hoping that all will go well and that I can easily sort out their fertility problems.

I return to the caveman principle often. Modern mankind is a mix of old behaviours and new technologies – some very new. The arrival of supermarkets and easily obtainable food is a very new event in the span of human history. Even growing food via agriculture is believed to be only 12,000 years old. Prior to that we lived a subsistence lifestyle. If my evolutionary reading is accurate, we inhabit a body that is not that different from the one formed two to three million years ago called *Homo erectus*.

I believe there are huge advantages in the differences between male and female behaviour. We should try as men to understand ourselves and our partners better, but that doesn't mean we have to meet in the middle. Testosterone and oestrogen are very different and so are men and women. Get your head around that thought – it will help you better understand the situation in which infertility places you. As well, it really helps in life in general.

Childlessness

This is a tough discussion. I looked after a couple in Ireland; he had a very low sperm count, and IVF was the only solution I could offer to help them. We tried to improve the sperm count with lifestyle modification to no avail. I knew they were not keen on IVF but that was all I could offer – that or using donor sperm.

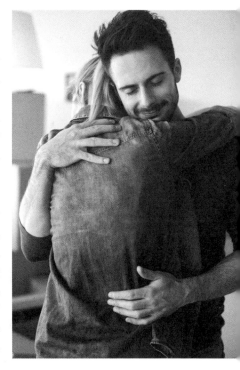

At some point they sensed my discomfort. 'Dr Greening, it's all right,' the man said. 'Some people don't get to have children. We'll be all right about that. We'll be a great uncle and a wonderful aunty.' Then he said, 'You are being too hard on yourself. You know it can't always work out. You can't help every couple get a child.'

I was stunned. In truth, that was *exactly* how I felt. Since then I have realised that some couples don't get to have children. Some don't try different options. Some try all the options and they do not work. The actual outcomes for infertility couples are hard to find, but perhaps 30 per cent may not achieve a child after treatment.

In the past childlessness was common. There were no treatments and, in general, a complete lack of understanding of why it happened. Couples coped with it in a world where answers were lacking in most areas.

In today's world where we have the answers to most questions, couples find this more difficult. It might happen to you as a couple. As I have said, men are 'fix it' creatures, but sometimes it cannot be fixed. Below are listed a few options for a childless couple.

 Adoption

Most couples have thought about this at least once during their infertility journey. In New Zealand in the 1960s adoption was quite common and most

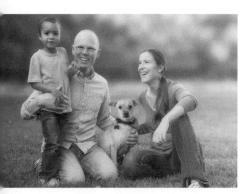

schools had several adopted children. From my reading, approximately 10 per cent of live births were to single mothers and well over 50 per cent of these were adopted out to non-related families. We all knew who they were, and it seemed perfectly normal to us. Adoption has changed over the decades, becoming far less common. Social welfare agencies and social ideals have changed. However, it may still be an option.

Research the available options either locally or overseas. There is quite a lot of information available on the internet.

TRAFFIC HAZARD	Multiple miscarriages and the road to adoption

Like most other young couples who have been married for several years, we started to excitedly turn our thoughts to starting a family. In preparation we purchased a larger house with sufficient bedrooms that would accommodate our plans.

We did not have too much problem with conceiving after a few months of trying. Our excitement was evident to all. After six or seven weeks my wife started to bleed and before we knew it my wife had miscarried. In looking back, I did not offer the emotional support that I should have to my wife rather in my typical positive self; I boldly proclaimed that we would probably have twins next. Again, we tried, and we had no significant issues with conceiving and after a few months we were pregnant.

After seven or eight weeks my wife started to bleed and again we miscarried. A similar story played out with pregnancy number three with another miscarriage. After the third miscarriage we enlisted the services of Dr Greening, who did significant tests on both of us. We hoped the tests would provide some reason for the miscarriages, which we could then address and have children, but the tests did not give any compelling reasons for why we could fall pregnant but not get past twelve weeks of pregnancy at most.

We continued to try, fall pregnant and lose the babies to miscarriage and after this occurred on six occasions we were in no place mentally or emotionally to try again. We were exhausted and beaten up and I felt helpless. I decided that this was our issue and that we would remain a team through these trials, that at times I felt would overwhelm me. I believe that we strengthened our relationship as we intentionally went through the battle as comrades together.

Having decided we could no longer contemplate building a family biologically, we turned our attention to adoption. We attended an intense information seminar, and before we knew it we had completed an application to start the very long process of adoption. This process was intrusive, slow and expensive, but I can say that after receiving the call from the New South Wales government that we had been allocated a four-month-old boy we could collect in two months, after the final paperwork was completed, was one of the happiest days of my life. A long few months later we travelled to Addis Ababa, Ethiopia, to collect our son. We were finally parents who had their son in their arms. It was the happiest of moments. My son, who at the time of writing is almost twelve, is amazing. He is strong socially ans academically and is a talented sportsman. He is my pride and joy.

As painful as the journey of creating a family through adoption was, I could not imagine our family without my son and I can truly say it was all worth it. I feel very blessed to have the family that I have.

Fostering

This is taking in a child at various ages for varying lengths of time. It is quite an undertaking and for novice couples can be a challenge – although a challenge that can be very fulfilling for both the couple and the child.

 Sperm donation

Sometimes men are born with no sperm production. It is the cards you have been dealt and it can take some time to get your head around. At some point the offer to use donated sperm will find its way into the doctor's discussion. You probably have thought about it already.

There are two ways to obtain sperm: either from a sperm bank that uses anonymous (unknown) donors or from someone you know, called a known donor. The discussion by the doctor will cover both possible options. Our unit has professionals who are experts in infertility counselling and I refer couples to them for an informed discussion. Obviously, this is an important discussion and many couples do not have a sperm donor they know. Who would? They might have a few potential candidates, but how to ask them? The counsellor can help with this.

Let's explore a known sperm donor scenario.

Tests confirm it is a sperm production problem and a testicular biopsy does not find any sperm. The discussion has yielded a brother who might be a candidate. The counsellor sees the couple and gives them information, so they can understand the sequence of events and requirements. Armed with the right information, the brother is approached. How?

My advice is that the two brothers meet alone and discuss the matter. Having a plan helps. Have some lines scripted so you know what you want to say:

'Jane and I have been seeing a doctor recently. You probably have already guessed, but we have had a fertility problem now for two years. Dr Greening has done tests and the problem is me: I was born without any sperm. He has suggested we will need a sperm donor and that a relative like a brother is a good possibility. I know this is a big topic to bring up and a lot to take in, but we would be grateful if you could consider our request. Take as much time as you need. I have all the information you might need and can get this to you. There is an excellent counsellor we have been to who can also answer all the questions you might have. It's a big topic, you're closer to me than anyone, and I thought of you first. Can we catch up in a week

or so and discuss? And if you don't want to do it we fully understand and there are other options we can use.'

That should get things started.

I would like to mention two points here you might never have considered.

Reverse the situation: let's say you have children and your brother approached you with the same question. What might be your answer? What would you think? What if he asked for a kidney as his had shut down and he was looking at lifelong dialysis? Look at the question from the other direction. It's a good strategy to consider a problem even if you don't have life experience of that issue.

Reverse the statistic: it's the same with statistics. If the chance of something is a percentage like 15 per cent then the remaining 85 per cent must be the opposite. If an IVF cycle has a 40 per cent chance of working, it must have a 60 per cent chance of not working. It is worth keeping in mind!

TRAFFIC HAZARD | Our sperm donor was a blessing

I was twenty-eight years of age, had been married for five years and, like most couples, ready to start a family. After a couple of months of trying my wife wasn't falling pregnant. She went to her local GP and had some routine tests that all came back good. The GP suggested I have a sperm count done. My test results were not what I expected – I had no sperm count. This was the start of my journey and a day I will never forget.

An appointment was made to see a fertility specialist and he advised me to have a testicular biopsy (small multiple incisions over both testes) to see if mature sperm could be found. We started our first IVF cycle.

Things did not go well. As confident as the doctor was, no mature sperm were found. He called this condition Sertoli cell-only syndrome. He advised us that with this type of condition there was nothing more he could do for us at this stage.

It all happened so fast it was like a big blur, and a very disappointing time in my life. We decided to get on with our lives. I decided to try herbal remedies and acupuncture – just to do something different and stay optimistic about everything.

(Cont.)

Five years passed, and we saw an advert in the local paper for a new infertility specialist in town. We made an appointment, and after several meetings we decided to give it another shot. A testicular biopsy was performed again, which meant another IVF cycle for my wife – we had nothing to lose. Results were not successful. Another heart-breaking moment for me, and for my wife – she was shattered.

All through this I was asked how I was coping with it all. How do you cope when you know you are the problem? I didn't smoke or drink and couldn't understand why this was happening to me or how I could have prevented it. No one could answer that. I was hurting. I had to stay strong and positive, not only for me but also for my wife.

We looked at our options and luckily for us we didn't have to try very hard. A special person who was part of our lives approached us and blessed us with a gift. He donated his sperm. Can you imagine what this meant to us? We had a chance of having what we wanted – a family!

After counselling sessions and more appointments, we were once again on another IVF cycle with the sperm donor. By the third attempt my wife fell pregnant, only to miscarry at seven weeks. We had gone from great highs to great lows.

On our fourth cycle we did it – a successful pregnancy and a beautiful baby girl. My princess was born in 2008. She is the best thing, apart from my wife, that could have happened to me.

The sperm donor was a blessing. It couldn't be my sperm, but it was his that brought my daughter into this world. In my eyes I will always look at her as if she were mine. To add to this note we took this journey once again and gave our daughter a brother.

For same-sex couples, they need to travel a different route to a heterosexual couple. For the women they will require intra-uterine insemination (IUI) or IVF with donor sperm.

Anonymous sperm donation is another option. Some infertility units have sperm banks and there are anonymous sperm banks. With an anonymous sperm bank a couple can access sperm from an unknown donor. The donor has produced sperm for a variety of reasons and allowed the unit to use it to assist couples produce a child. It is an amazing gift.

Sperm banks are extremely well organised. The process involves a male deciding to be a donor. He contacts the unit. He is screened to see if he complies with all the regulations of the unit and the law. Next, he will be tested; obviously a semen analysis and various other tests are performed. This check is for infectious diseases such as hepatitis B, hepatitis C and HIV as well as other viruses. A genetic test is done to confirm that there are no significant abnormalities such as cystic fibrosis. Medical and family histories are taken to exclude any potential inheritable diseases. This takes some time. Once all is completed and the donor is approved, he will produce the semen, which is stored at -196°C (-320°F) in liquid nitrogen. Information regarding the sperm donor is taken. His semen analysis may be normal or even abnormal with low count or motility. Both are acceptable to a sperm bank once thoroughly checked. This donor's sperm is only suitable for use in IVF and not for IUI.

The infertile couple may then approach the sperm bank for sperm. If the female partner is considered to have no or few factors contributing to infertility the option of IUI may be offered. IUI with normal sperm has a reasonable pregnancy rate per attempt and is very much female age dependent.

For example, if the female partner is aged thirty then IUI is a reasonable option. If she is aged thirty-seven, IVF using donor sperm may offer advantages. It has a better pregnancy rate per try but, more importantly, it can potentially result in frozen embryos. If the couple try IUI and it works, great! But for an attempt at baby number two the woman will be close to forty and her biological clock has reduced her fertility significantly. Those frozen embryos will be important.

TRAFFIC HAZARD | Some rules that may help during sperm donation

Rule one. Don't talk too much or try to fix it. Acknowledge the emotions. Most of your emotions may be a reaction to her emotions, or vice versa.

Rule two. Think about how to deal with it. Read something about it or get advice – the counsellor you met about infertility can help.

Rule three. Do something. Buy a book on sperm donation or print out some information from the internet. Make time to talk about it. Mention that you are different – yin and yang – and that's a good thing. Bringing it up will really help you see the issues from the other point of view.

(Cont.)

> I have a few couples that are both yin or both yang. This is always difficult. Either they both are totally stressed about the infertility problems, or they can't seem to deal with them at all and avoid them. A yin and yang couple cover a wider range of human personality and behaviours. That range is a good thing.

IUI is the most common method used if acceptable to the doctor and couple after discussion. The couple then develop a management plan with the doctor. For example, they might decide they are going to attempt six cycles of IUI during the woman's natural cycle. The couple attend the sperm bank and get the details of how the system works. The process is outlined, donors are matched to the couple and each unit follows certain rules and legalities. The donor is usually racially matched to start with, then the couple can review potential characteristics of the donors. They may both be academics with PhD qualifications and looking for that. They may be manual labourers or currently unemployed. Infertility is not a disease that targets any single group; male factor problems are quite random. Having narrowed down potential donors, a decision must be made as to which one to use.

A donor is chosen. He will remain the couple's donor for all attempts and, if successful, for further attempts at siblings for child number one. That way, the children all have the same genetic background.

The female cycle is tracked, and ovulation dates confirmed. The IUI procedure is scheduled and the usual paperwork is finalised. You both arrive (*both!*) on the day and the simple procedure of injecting a specially prepared sample of sperm is done, usually quickly and easily.

You go off to do your thing and your partner follows the advice of the clinic: rest or go back to work. Then you wait to see if a pregnancy occurs. This can be repeated up to six times, taking around six months.

In most situations an ongoing pregnancy occurs, occasionally a miscarriage. Infertility patients who conceive also miscarry like the fertile group. It hurts.

If six cycles or so do not work, the doctor will see you to discuss options – further cycles or IVF.

Legal and ethical requirements

Donor sperm and egg treatment (and particularly surrogacy) are very carefully regulated in most countries. Even within a country, different states can have different laws or requirements. It is beyond the scope of this book to cover this, but your local reproductive unit should be able to provide the legal and ethical requirements.

Ethically there are many ways to look at donation. Many groups have their own approaches to these treatments, for example, the use of donated sperm or eggs is forbidden in Islam. Couples should make their own decisions with as much information as they can that pertains to them. Ultimately, final decisions will have personal, ethical and legal components to them.

Egg donation

Occasionally a couple require a donor egg for multiple reasons. the woman has none, premature menopause, or repeated IVF failure. Mostly it is a female age issue and the egg quality is the problem. If aged over forty, egg donation may become an alternative if IVF is failing or if egg quality is poor. This changes the game significantly. Young donated eggs give a couple excellent success rates. Anonymous egg donors in Spain are typically around twenty-three years of age and Spain is a significant European source of donor eggs, just like Denmark is the leading source of anonymous donor sperm.

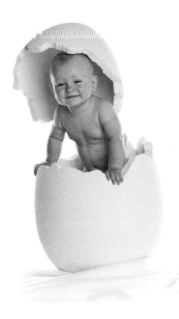

Once again, the options are a known donor or an unknown (anonymous) donor. A known donor may include a relative, friend or colleague. Some couples advertise for a donor and develop a relationship with them with the aim of using them as a donor.

Many countries allow donors to be paid, but in Australia commercial egg donation is not allowed by law. Neither is commercial sperm donation. Consequently, egg donation in Australia is difficult (sperm donation is less so). Finding your own donor can be hard – a known donor needs to be young, preferably younger than thirty-eight, sure she wants to do it and healthy. She needs to be screened by a counsellor to be sure she is a viable candidate.

The next step is to see the doctor and set up the egg donation cycle. The doctor will explain. If travelling to another country such as Spain, Greece, South Africa or the United States the doctors will help co-ordinate the process.

Costs vary, and you need to do some research.

I won't go into this in depth again but essentially the egg donor goes through a stimulated IVF cycle, your female partner has treatment to get her cycle into synchronicity with the donor, and you travel along to provide the sperm on the day of egg collection. Three to five days after egg collection the embryo is transferred back into your partner and if it succeeds she has a nine month pregnancy. It's different to sperm donation as your partner gets to carry the pregnancy. It might not be her egg, but it is *her* pregnancy. Remaining embryos are frozen for future potential use.

Same-sex couples will require an egg donor. Male same-sex couples will also require a surrogate to carry the pregnancy. For them much is involved but the principles of donation are the same.

TRAFFIC HAZARD — Donation: who do you tell?

My advice is to tell only a few about the egg or sperm donation. A few people will understand but many won't. Counsellors can advise you. I often suggest that couples take an overseas 'holiday' (that is, do an IVF donor egg cycle). Surprisingly, they come home pregnant after years of trying to conceive. Incredible! Amazing!

Most people don't need to know an egg donor was involved: you decide what to do. Maybe later in life you can explain it, but it really can be difficult. People don't always understand when they have two or three kids made the easy way. Perhaps in years to come people in societies will be more accepting of egg and sperm donation or surrogacy, but I find it can be difficult for a couple if others make comments that hurt them, and it may hurt your relationship with them.

Once again, discuss it together and formulate a plan on how to deal with this issue.

Facilitators

When it comes to egg donation, it can be useful to use a reproductive facilitator. I discovered one many years ago and refer patients to her. A former nurse in an IVF unit, she arranges egg donations in Europe for overseas couples. She finds them a unit, be it in Spain or Greece or elsewhere. She liaises with your doctor then the donor IVF/IUI unit, to determine what exactly the donor unit requires from the couple: blood tests, scans and so forth. She even books flights and accommodation and makes the couple's road to egg donation as straightforward as she can. See the Resources section for contact details (www. ivftreatmentabroad.com).

I have used Ruth Pellow for over a decade and I'm sure there are many others. They make the difficult process simpler, reduce the stress of overseas donation and have a track record. My patients universally have found the facilitation process helps them, enormously.

 ## Surrogacy

Occasionally the woman cannot carry a pregnancy due to various causes. She may have congenital absence of the uterus (called Mayer-Rokitansky Kuster Hauser syndrome. I guess all four discovered it at once) or has required a hysterectomy for a serious reason. She may have Asherman's syndrome, where the uterine cavity is damaged. Two patients I dealt with had lost their uterus due to motor vehicle accidents.

A surrogate will offer to carry the pregnancy for the couple. The couple must go through IVF and make embryos, then the female surrogate has the embryo transferred to her uterus. If she falls pregnant, she carries the foetus to term and the commissioning couple adopt the baby back. Genetically it is theirs even though the kind surrogate has incubated the embryo through to birth. It's a complicated but hugely fulfilling process that I have been fortunate to be part of a few times, including being their obstetrician. Most larger IVF units have this available.

Be aware this is a very complicated and long road with many legal and ethical requirements. Ultimately, however, it is simply extraordinary to be able to do this and to be a part of it. The few I have done have been an amazing part of my own medical journey.

 ## Uterine transplant

In this very new surgical procedure a healthy donated uterus is transplanted into a recipient female whose own uterus may have been damaged or absent from birth. The method was developed at the University of Gothenburg by a Swedish team under Dr Mats Brännström. I was at an American Society for Reproductive Medicine conference in Honolulu in 2014 when Mats presented the results of his twenty years of work; he received a standing ovation.

It is a new procedure, but it has now arrived on the scene. Watch this space.

Complementary and alternative medical treatments

The original version of this book had a full chapter on complementary and alternative treatments (CAM), but to keep what you're holding to a readable size it had to go. From a research perspective, medically there is very little to support these methods despite all the information you may read or be told. If there was evidence to support CAM, REI/OBGYN, doctors would make use of it, I promise you. That said, you can choose whatever path you wish for treatments. I suggest you look at the Cochrane database section on CAM at www.cam.cochrane.org. It covers a huge amount of research and not just reproductive CAMs.

ROUGH SURFACE	Summary

- Sometimes your life situation means you must choose a different route to get to your planned destination, to choose *other options*. You have to follow a different route on the road map and take the roads less travelled.
- That might be egg or sperm donation or even surrogacy, something you probably never considered early on in your relationship. The same goes for adopting or fostering a child.
- Other options may in fact be the only way forward and childlessness is one of the options you may choose. Some couples decide their journey is going to be just their own and drive a road together forever. They are a family of two.
- There are always other options that will present themselves to you on this fertility journey. You expect to drive to a certain destination and find you must take a completely alternative route. You must include other passengers if you take the donor option; they will leave when you arrive at your destination and will give you a truly amazing gift: a baby. I have seen this many times. An organ donation is one thing but donating eggs or sperm to make a baby is something completely different.

- You might not arrive where you hoped. You might not have a biological child, but the two of you got in that car and you drove.
- You might end up back at square one – just the two of you – but you'll have had an incredible trip with many different twists and turns. Other people might hop in the car to help carry your baby or donate an egg or sperm.
- As Randy Pausch said, 'It's not about the cards you're dealt, but how you play the hand.'

CHAPTER 17

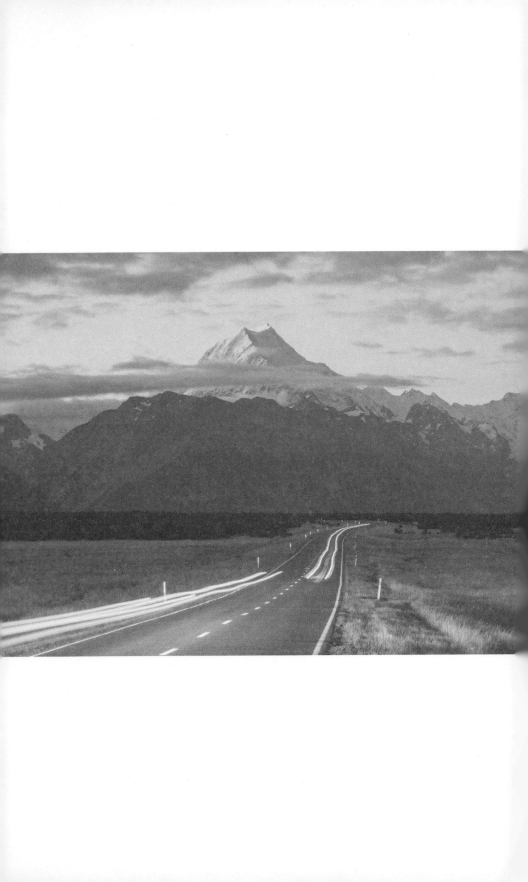

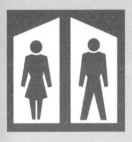

The journey onwards

I hope this book has been a useful and supportive guide on your journey, a road map for each couple reading it. Every couple starts from a position of concern about infertility but each must reach their own destination, and there is no guarantee as to what that will look like.

I wrote this book to help couples on that journey, and particularly to assist the men to share the driving.

Fertility is assumed – men and women assume they will be fine and have no problems conceiving. Unfortunately, one in six couples has problems conceiving. One in six!

You will recall that primary infertility means twelve months of trying to conceive with no previous pregnancies of any sort. Secondary infertility, on the other hand, is just six months of infertility with a previous pregnancy, be it a live birth, miscarriage, ectopic (tubal) pregnancy, a termination or a biochemical pregnancy.

Male factors are responsible for 30 to 40 per cent of infertility problems. Invariably, that's a sperm issue. Getting a semen analysis is the first step for a man.

You have been introduced to the anatomy and functioning of men and women, where you came from, and how that tiny Y chromosome had so many profound effects on you and the X chromosome on your partner. Hopefully, you have come to understand some of the complexities of our incredible reproductive systems. Your understanding of your amazing female partner should have been enhanced; her side of the reproductive process is far more complex than yours.

You now know the top five requirements for fertility:

- **Sperm:** necessary and usually around 30 to 40 per cent of the problem.
- **Ovulation:** ovulation day is approximately the length of the menstrual cycle minus fourteen days. Ovulation disorders like polycystic ovary syndrome make up 25 per cent of couple fertility problems.
- **Sex:** it's important to know the facts and equally important to understand how to make your sex life work again, especially if you're dealing with the stress of infertility.
- **Tubes:** the fallopian tubes need to be open so that the sperm and egg can meet. Problems in this area can be the cause of up to 20 to 25 per cent of infertility issues.
- **Timing:** If all the four factors above are normal, you still need to get your timing right for sex to conceive. Having sex during ovulation is not rocket science! Remember my advice: to lower the chance of sperm DNA damage and increase your chances of a successful conception have sex for seven days in a row, with ovulation day around day five.

There is no way around the age factor, especially your partner's age. Knowing her eggs are as old as her and that they have less fertility potential as they pass thirty-six years of age is useful information. While getting the anti-Müllerian hormone ovarian-reserve test is not routinely recommended, it can be helpful. Age is a huge factor, so consider it before deciding on children. Discuss it openly.

And if you are getting older get a medical check-up: you get your car serviced regularly! If you are going to be a father your children deserve a healthy parent.

Think about your lifestyle. Smoking, the consumption of alcohol, weight and age (again) are all factors in infertility. Take a good hard look at your lifestyle to identify areas you could improve. Don't just think about it, do it. My grandfather Charlie Greening, who fought in World War I in the trenches, used to say: 'You can wish in one hand and spit in the other, and at the end of the day you will have a hand full of spit.' He didn't believe in wishes, he believed in doing something positive.

Don't just sit there: do something about it!

You're on this road trip as a team, you and your partner. Honour that and all it means.

Specialists like me are in this business because we want to help you achieve your dream of starting a family. But there are no guarantees, and as much as medicine continues to advance there probably never will be.

Perhaps your journey will see you set out as two and return with a baby on the way, achieved naturally, through assisted reproduction, with donated egg or sperm or by using a surrogate. Perhaps you will take a different route to creating a family – adopting or fostering. Or perhaps you will find you have to let that dream go and find another way to share your love, becoming the world's best aunty and uncle.

Whatever your destination, I hope you find contentment.

David Greening

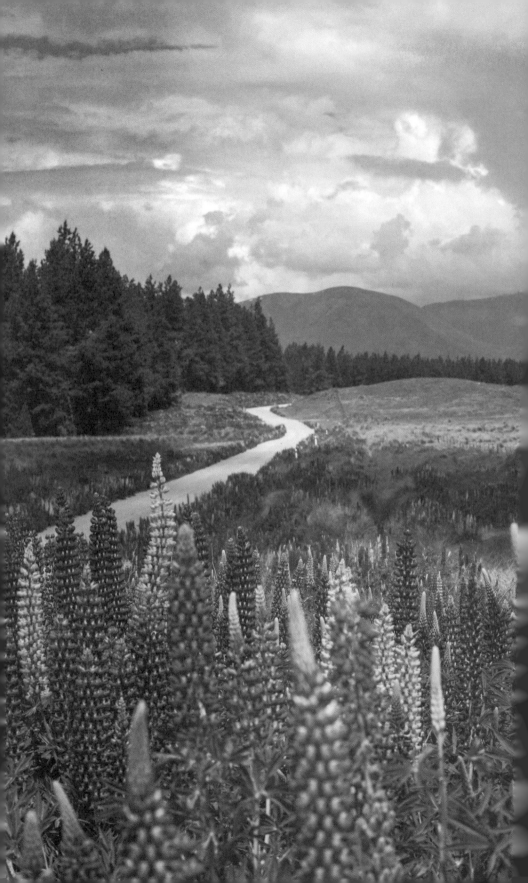

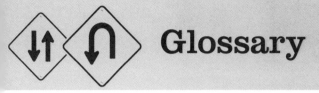

Glossary

abortion	Miscarriage before twenty weeks of pregnancy. May be spontaneous, incomplete, therapeutic, social, threatened or missed.
adhesion	Scar tissue formed from disease or trauma. Common with endometriosis, or after previous surgery.
adrenal gland	Two glands found on top of the kidneys that make several hormones such as dehydroepiandrosterone (DHEA).
amenorrhoea	The lack of a female period occurring for six months or more. 'Primary' means never and 'secondary' means once had periods but they have now stopped for six months.
androgens	Male hormones that masculinise, for example, testosterone, androstenedione. Mostly produced in the testes but there are some in the adrenal glands. Often raised in females with PCOS.
andrologist	A specialist doctor who deals with male fertility and hormones.
anovulation	Absence of ovulation; 'an' means lack of.
anti-Müllerian hormone (AMH)	This reflects the number of eggs in the ovaries. Known as the egg timer or ovarian-reserve test. Usually decreases with female age. High in PCOS.
artificial insemination	The injection of sperm, be it a partner's or donor sperm, into the vagina/cervix.
Asherman's syndrome	A condition of scar tissue inside the uterus.

aspiration	Suctioning with a needle. Egg aspiration is a standard IVF technique.
assisted reproductive technologies (ART)	Includes IVF, IUI, GIFT.
asthenoteratozoospermia	Low motility and poor-shaped sperm.
asthenozoospermia	Sperm with low motility.
azoospermia	The absence of sperm in an ejaculation, due to non-production or a blockage.
baby	A small, often noisy, smelly infant human of the genus *Homo sapiens*. Often has no idea of the difficulty the adult parents had to achieve and as a teenager won't care anyway.
basal body temperature (BBT)	Taken mid-cycle to see if ovulation may have occurred; usually a small rise is seen.
beta HCG	The pregnancy hormone tested for through a blood or urine test.
bicornuate uterus	One of the congenital uterine shapes that may affect pregnancy.
blastocyst	The five-day-old embryo that implants in the uterus; also the most common IVF embryo transferred. Refers to an embryo that has blastulated, that is, expanded itself with fluid within which is the inner cell mass. This becomes the foetus and is surrounded by the trophectoderm, which becomes the placenta and membranes.
blighted ovum	A miscarriage. The pregnancy sac is seen but there is no embryo within.
cervix	The lower end of the uterus. Pap smears are taken from this.
chromosome	The structure that contains our genes: Twenty-three per sperm or egg; forty-six per most human cells.
clinical pregnancy	An ultrasound-proven early pregnancy with a foetal heartbeat.
clomid	Clomiphene citrate, a widely used ovulation drug. Usually taken orally on day two to six of a female cycle, to stimulate ovulation.

congenital bilateral absence of the vas deferens (CBAVD)	No vas develops; azoospermic, but sperm are present in the testes. Sometimes associated with the cystic fibrosis gene.
contraceptive	A device or drug to suppress female or male fertility.
corpus luteum	The follicle that the egg was in becomes a cyst known as a corpus luteum; it secretes progesterone to help implantation and support the early pregnancy.
cryopreservation	Freezing eggs, sperm or embryos to preserve them during ART. Mostly achieved through a process called vitrification.
Cushing's syndrome	Named after Harvey Cushing, who found excess cortisol from the adrenal gland. Can affect fertility as a cause of PCOS.
cycle	Either a natural monthly menstrual cycle in a female or an ART cycle attempt.
cyst	A sac; in the ovary called an ovarian cyst.
dehydroepi-androsterone sulphate (DHEAS)	An adrenal androgen, and excess of which can affect fertility. Blood tests diagnose this. Associated with excess hair growth and acne.
diagnostic	To help diagnose a condition or problem.
dilatation and curettage (D&C)	The term for dilate and curette. A surgical procedure to dilate the cervix and remove the lining of the uterus. Either diagnostic or after miscarriage.
dildo	An artificial mechanical penis of various shapes to assist during sex. Best hidden well in case of unforeseen embarrassment when the parents-in-law find it.
dodo	A sad now extinct bird once found on Madagascar. Supposedly exceedingly dumb and often the term is now used for the male of the human species by frustrated partners. Ostrich is also often used in the same context.
donor	Someone who donates tissue, be it sperm, eggs or embryos (or body parts).
donor insemination (DI)	Injecting a donor's sperm into the cervix.

dysfunctional uterine bleeding (DUB)	Often seen with PCOS, it has an abnormal cycle length.
ectopic pregnancy	The fertilised egg implants in the fallopian tube or elsewhere in the pelvis. Can be a serious medical emergency if it bleeds.
egg	The female egg or oocyte, produced approximately monthly with the aim of being fertilised by a male sperm to produce an embryo. Contains only twenty-three chromosomes instead of a normal body cell's forty-six. The largest human cell. Lives approximately twenty-four hours unless fertilised or frozen during ART.
ejaculation	The act of expelling semen. Highly regarded by the male species.
embryo	The first eight weeks of a human foetus.
embryo transfer	During IVF the transfer of an embryo from the lab into the female uterus.
endocrine	The hormones made in the body. A reproductive endocrine is the hormone as it pertains to fertility.
endometrial biopsy	One of the tests for the structure and functionality of the endometrium, including the level of natural killer cells.
endometriosis	A disease where the endometrium grows in abnormal places such as the ovary or pelvis. Adenomyosis is a version of this where the endometrium grows in the muscular wall of the uterus called the myometrium.
endometrium	The lining of the uterus designed for implantation of a human embryo.
epididymis	The storage area after the testes have made the sperm. One area where sperm DNA damage can occur.
estrogen	*See* **oestrogen**.
ethics committee	An independent multi-disciplinary team of experts to make decisions regarding ethical matters as part of ART. Bioethics is the 'understanding of the moral life'; ethics committees assess the morality of decisions with regard to patients.

fallopian tubes	The tubes connected to the uterus up which the sperm swim and down which the egg comes from the ovary. Fertilisation occurs in the tube and the embryo migrates down the tube into the uterine cavity.
Femara (letrozole)	A widely used ovulation drug.
fertilisation	The joining of sperm and egg.
fertility specialist	Usually an OBGYN who has trained in the field of reproductive endocrinology and infertility REI and requires extra training after obgyn.
fibroid	A common benign (not cancerous) tumour of the wall (myometrium) of the uterus. Also called a myoma; rarely malignant. May be on the outside (sub-serosal), in the wall (intra-mural) or indent the uterine cavity (sub-mucous).
foetus	A human embryo from eight weeks on until delivery. Before that it is known as an embryo.
folic acid	B group vitamin also called folate. The only proven vitamin to reduce spina bifida. Various recommended doses depending on different countries.
follicle	The small sac-like structure within which the female egg grows. Releases the egg down the fallopian tube or is aspirated during IVF to collect the egg.
follicle-stimulating hormone (FSH)	A hormone made in the pituitary gland in the brain that acts on the ovary to stimulate the growth of a follicle and therefore egg. Synthetic FSH is used during ART to grow follicles and is given as a daily injection.
follicular tracking	Serial ultrasound scans and blood tests to track a female cycle to determine ovulation. It is used both during natural and ART cycles.
fragile X syndrome	A sex-linked chromosomal disorder. Causes male mental retardation if a male foetus inherits the gene on the X chromosome. Females are carriers. Linked to premature ovarian insufficiency, that is, premature menopause in female carriers.

gamete	A mature human sex cell, that is, a sperm or an egg. Has twenty-three human cell chromosomes, compared to somatic (body) cells with forty-six chromosomes.
gene	The package of inherited DNA that codes for proteins. Humans have approximately 31,000 genes, which are individual small parts of the complete architectural design to build a human.
gonad	The glands that produce sex cells. Ovaries in a female and testes in the male.
gonadotropin	A hormone that switches on the ovary or testes (the gonads), for example, FSH, LH.
gonadotropin-releasing hormone (GnRH)	The hypothalamus hormone that acts on the pituitary to produce gonadotropins. Inhibited during IVF to stop ovulation.
haploid	A cell with twenty-three chromosomes, such as an egg or sperm.
hirsutism	Excess body hair, seen in PCOS due to excess androgens, that is, male hormones
hormonal assay	Blood tests to measure hormones like FSH, LH and testosterone.
hormones	Chemicals produced in a gland that have effects somewhere else in the body.
human chorionic gonadotropin (HCG)	The pregnancy hormone produced by the early embryo. Its role is to maintain early progesterone levels. HCG is the most sought-after hormone in the fertility world.
hyperinsulinemia	Over-production of insulin with possible associated effects including PCOS, high blood pressure, diabetes, high cholesterol, weight gain. Also called metabolic syndrome or syndrome X.
hyperthyroidism	The condition of excess thyroxine production by the thyroid gland, which can affect ovulation.
hypothyroidism	The condition of reduced thyroxine production. Slows metabolism and affects fertility.
hyperprolactinaemia	Excess levels of prolactin due to a gland in the pituitary gland called a prolactinoma.

hysterosalpingo-contrast-sonography (HyCoSY)	An ultrasound procedure to inject dye through the cervix and then ultrasound is used to assess the uterine cavity and tubal function. A test for tubal patency and for the shape of the uterus.
hysterosalpingogram (HSG)	An X-ray version of HyCoSy with the same principle.
hysteroscopy	A surgical procedure to use a 5 mm (0.2 in) telescope to look inside the uterus. Most are done under general anaesthetic, although some are done in offices.
implantation	The process of an embryo embedding itself in the endometrium of the uterus and developing
impotence	The inability of a male to have erections. Either psychological or physiological. Increasing problem with increasing length of infertility.
infertility	The inability to conceive after twelve months of trying and no previous pregnancies. If a previous pregnancy, then the inability to conceive after six months of trying.
insemination	The injection of sperm into a female uterus to aid in achieving a pregnancy.
intracytoplasmic sperm injection (ICSI)	A process during IVF of injecting a single sperm into a single egg where the male semen analysis has shown low sperm count, motility or morphology or all three. Approximately 50 per cent or more of IVF worldwide uses the ICSI technique.
intra-uterine insemination (IUI)	Injection of semen by catheter into the female uterus. This can be the partner's semen or donor semen.
in vitro fertilisation (IVF)	First began in 1978 and involves the taking of sperm and eggs out of the body to fertilise them, growing the embryo for three to five days then transferring the embryo back to the uterus. Compared to in vivo fertilisation, which occurs inside the body naturally.
karyotype	A test that displays the chromosomes. Males are 46XY and females 46XX. Abnormalities may be found and termed aneuploid; normal is termed euploid.

Klinefelter syndrome	A condition of an extra X chromosome 47, XXY called trisomy. Linked to either no sperm (azoospermia) or sometimes low sperm numbers (oligospermia).
laparoscopy	Keyhole surgery to allow a small telescope to see inside the abdomen and pelvis. Requires a general anaesthetic and may be a diagnostic procedure to just look or an operative procedure to remove endometriosis, fibroids and/or adhesions.
laparotomy	A surgical procedure that opens the abdomen or pelvis. For example, microsurgery to repair fallopian tubes is done as an open procedure. Larger fibroids, bowel surgery and caesarean section are all open procedures.
last menstrual period (LMP)	The first day of proper full bleeding is denoted day one of that menstrual cycle.
Leydig cells	Cells in the testes that produce male hormone-like testosterone. Stimulated by the LH hormone from the pituitary gland.
luteal phase	A phase in the female cycle after ovulation is called the luteal phase. The follicle remains as the corpus luteum and produces progesterone, which rises to support a pregnancy if it occurs. HCG from the embryo rescues the corpus luteum, which then vastly increases progesterone production until around twelve weeks, when the placenta takes over.
luteinising hormone (LH)	Has two functions. Is released by the pituitary in females to stimulate the ovary to ovulate the egg by a huge surge in hormone, usually mid menstrual cycle. In men it stimulates the testes to produce testosterone.
male factor infertility	The male as the cause of infertility accounts for approximately 30 to 40 per cent of causes. This may be either a sperm issue or performance issue.
menopause	The cessation of periods as the egg supply in the ovary runs out. Occurs at an average age of fifty-one. When aged younger than forty it denotes premature menopause, known as premature ovarian insufficiency.

menorrhagia	Heavy menstrual bleeding; often the cause of anaemia.
menses	A period. Denotes the shedding of the endometrium on a cyclic monthly timeframe if a pregnancy does not occur. Usually commences between ages twelve and sixteen.
microsurgery	Surgery using a microscope. Examples are commonly vasectomy or tubal ligation reversal. It is one of my favourite types of surgery.
miscarriage	Spontaneous loss of a pregnancy before twenty weeks. The miscarriage rate is female age dependent. Habitual or recurrent miscarriage refers to three miscarriages in succession and is routinely investigated.
mittelschmerz	German for mid-cycle ovulation pain. Can be normal or can mean endometriosis.
mosaicism	Where the karyotype is mixed and denoted by percentages. The lab counts the different type of cells. *See also* **Turner syndrome.**
Müllerian anomalies	Congenital abnormal development of the Müllerian structure, which makes the uterus tubes and vagina. For example, uterine didelphys, or two uteri.
mumps	Infection of the parotid gland in the neck. May spread to the testes, causing mumps orchitis (a cause of azoospermia and sterility).
myomectomy	Surgical procedure to remove fibroid/s. Either done using a laparoscope or as an open procedure if the fibroid is large.
natural killer cells	Immuno-surveillance cells found throughout the body but high in the endometrium. Excess levels may contribute to implantation dysfunction or to miscarriage. Assessed by ether a blood test or endometrial biopsy.
necrospermia	Sperm that are dead.

oestrogen	The female hormone produced by the ovary. It has multiple functions, principally the development of female sexual characteristics. Various forms are oestradiol, oestrone, oestriol.
oligoasthenoterato-zoospermia	Low sperm count, motility and shape.
oligomenorrhea	Menstrual periods that occur less frequently than normal.
oligospermia	Low sperm numbers in an ejaculation.
oocyte	The human female egg from the ovary. Has a haploid number of chromosomes (twenty-three). The largest human cell, three thousand times larger than a sperm. Stored in the female foetal ovary and depleted as each ovulation occurs, as opposed to sperm, which are continually being made. Referred to as a gamete.
orchitis	Infection of the testes. Mumps orchitis may cause sterility by damaging the sperm-producing cells.
ovarian failure	The condition where the ovary no longer responds to FSH hormone. Associated with an elevated FSH.
ovarian hyperstimulation syndrome (OHSS)	Over-stimulation of the ovaries due to the IVF trigger injection. A cascade of chemicals starts that leads to massive fluid accumulation in the abdomen or lungs with a risk of blood clots. Can be life threatening.
ovary	The female gonad gland in the pelvis that produces eggs (oocytes) and female hormones oestrogen and progesterone.
ovulation	The release of the egg from the ovary.
ovulation induction	The use of drugs to induce the ovary to ovulate an egg. Common drugs include clomiphene citrate (Clomid), letrozole (Femara) tablets or injections of FSH.

Pap smear	A test to detect abnormal precancerous/cancerous cells of the cervix. Routinely done bi- or tri-annually depending on the country.
pelvic inflammatory disease (PID)	Infection of the fallopian tubes and pelvis commonly caused by chlamydia or gonorrhoea (sexually transmitted diseases), which can damage the fallopian tubes and cause infertility and/or raise the risk of an ectopic pregnancy.
penis	The awesome external male sexual organ. Has dual function to urinate through and to pass semen into the female vagina. Size range is considerable; the average is 13 cm (5 in) when erect.
pituitary gland	A master gland in the brain. Produces the reproductive hormones FSH and LH and prolactin as well as thyroid-stimulating hormone, growth hormone and a lot more. Fundamental to egg production and ovulation as well as sperm production.
polycystic ovarian syndrome (PCOS)	Females with polycystic ovaries (less than twelve per ovary) have irregular cycles, increased male hormones, acne and increased hair production as well as infertility. Commonly associated with hyperinsulinemia.
pre-implantation genetic diagnosis (PGD)	An IVF procedure in which cells are biopsied from an embryo then tested for genetic condition; unaffected embryos are then used. Specific genetic conditions can be diagnosed such as cystic fibrosis, or embryo screening tests look for chromosomal anomalies. Sometimes called pre-implantation genetic screening.
primary infertility	Never previously pregnant and been trying for twelve months.

progesterone	The hormone made from the follicle that becomes the corpus luteum. Supports the early pregnancy and has an immunological mechanism to allow the embryo to implant and remain.
prostate gland	Produces prostate fluid, which makes up part of semen. Protects the early sperm from the vaginal fluids. Prostate-specific antigen (PSA) dissolves the initial semen clot to allow it to race up the cervix. High PSA may indicate prostate cancer. More men die each year from prostate cancer than do females from breast cancer.
recurrent pregnancy loss	Refers to two or commonly three successive losses of a pregnancy.
reproductive endocrinology and infertility (REI)	Sub-specialty within obstetrics and gynaecology that requires advanced training. In Australia, directors of fertility units must have this extra qualification.
retrograde ejaculation	Semen ejaculates backwards into the bladder from the urethra, usually due to either a neurological disorder or previous pelvic trauma. Semen can be found in urine. It is rare.
Rhesus factor	Denotes the positive or negative component of a blood group. Blood groups are O, A, B or AB. Rhesus refers to the D antigen. Lack of D denotes a negative blood group; if D is found it denotes a positive. If a mother is Rhesus negative and the foetus is positive (from the positive father) there may be pregnancy issues.
rubella	German measles. All pre-pregnant women should be vaccinated against this condition to create immunity.
salpingectomy	Surgical removal of the fallopian tube. Common after an ectopic pregnancy.
scrotum	The ball sac found below the penis within which are the testes.

secondary infertility	Infertility after previous pregnancies as opposed to primary infertility, where no previous pregnancy has ever occurred.
secondary sexual	The development at puberty of characteristics associated with maturity such characteristics as breasts and beards; distinguishes females from males.
semen	The fluid within which is the sperm. Includes prostate fluid and fructose.
semen analysis	Examination under a microscope of sperm for count, motility and shape. Sperm are the taxi to take the sperm DNA to meet the female egg DNA.
sperm bank	Frozen sperm is kept for use during artificial insemination or IVF. Anonymous donors have contributed sperm under strict criteria and regulations.
sperm DNA damage	Examination of sperm to assess DNA damage. DNA is the passenger component of the sperm (the taxi). A more modern test and not all units assess this. Tests include the tunnel assay, comet assay and SCSA assay. All measure the DNA strand breakage rate.
sperm wash	A procedure prior to using the sperm to wash off any residual chemicals or toxins.
sterility	A form of infertility but denotes the complete inability to conceive, for example, complete azoospermia requiring a sperm donor or premature ovarian failure.
steroids	Hormones made originally from cholesterol that cover the spectrum from oestrogen to testosterone. Artificial steroids include prednisolone, used to reduce natural killer cells, through to anabolic steroids, used in gyms to gain muscle mass such as testosterone.
superovulation	Fertility treatment to ovulate more than a single egg. IVF cycles can routinely produce up to fifteen eggs.

surrogacy	Where one female receives an embryo created by the commissioning couple and acts as a recipient, then carries the pregnancy through to delivery for the couple. The baby is returned to the commissioning couple under strict regulatory and legal arrangements. Either a commercial arrangement or altruistic.
testes	The male gonad reproductive gland that produces sperm and testosterone. Found beneath the penis in a ball sac.
testicular biopsy	Various methods to biopsy the testes to get sperm if there is an obstruction or low production. An open biopsy, needle biopsy or epididymal aspiration by needle.
testosterone	Male hormone produced by the testes and the main determinant of masculinisation for a male. Females have a small amount. In the uterus it masculinises the male 46XY foetus. In the testes the sperm is exposed to high levels. A steroid that can be used to supplement men with low levels or as a muscle-building steroid.
transvaginal oocyte retrieval (TVOR)	The technical term of an IVF egg collection.
tubal ligation	A permanent contraceptive surgical procedure to cut or clip the fallopian tubes. Performed by laparoscope.
Turner syndrome	A condition of lacking one of the normal X chromosomes, making the female 45X(0). True Turners 45X(0) have no ovaries, experience no puberty and are sterile. Requires a reproductive specialist to treat to achieve puberty. Some are Turner mosaics 45X/46XX and may have small functioning ovaries.
ultrasound	Uses high frequency sound waves to image the internal organs, either as an abdominal probe or vaginal probe. IVF egg collections are done using ultrasound.

unexplained infertility   Where basic infertility investigation fails to find a cause for a couple's infertility when semen analysis, tubal dye studies, ovulation tests and ultrasound are all normal and regular sex is taking place. Further investigations such as laparoscopy or genetic or immunological tests may discover the reason.

urethra   The tube in the penis that urine flows along from the bladder. Joined by the vas deferens from the testes.

uterus   The muscular female organ that the embryo implants into and grows through to term. Delivers the baby by a contractile process called labour.

vaginal probe   A standard ultrasound method of visualising female organs such as the uterus, ovaries and surrounding structures as well as an early pregnancy.

vaginitis   Inflammation of the vagina due to infection or chemical, for example, candidiasis (thrush).

varicocele   Large varicose veins found in the scrotum.

vas deferens   The tube that sperm swim along from the testes to join the urethra. Congenitally absent in CBAVD.

vasectomy   Cutting the vas deferens for permanent contraception.

vasectomy reversal   Microsurgery to repair the vasectomy and restore natural fertility.

venereal disease   Sexually transmitted infection including chlamydia, gonorrhoea and syphilis; may cause infertility.

zygote   The initial stage after an egg and sperm fertilise. The zygote becomes a morula then a blastocyst and finally an embryo.

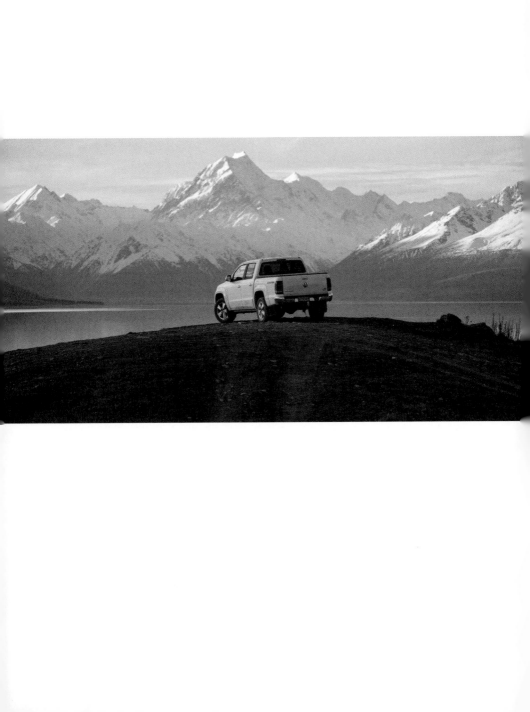

Resources

There are many resources for infertile couples and individuals that are available in many countries; in fact, a staggeringly large amount. You should do your own research to find these, although I include a few here.

Australia

- Fertility Society of Australia (www.fertilitysociety.com.au). This is a combined group containing doctors, nurses, scientists and counsellors that has been a huge success in Australia. Look up the guidelines under patient information.
- Access Australia (www.access.org.au). A national support network for patients that is our pre-eminent patient support and information group. Access is a strong advocate for the infertile with information, support and referrals.
- Donor Conception Support Network (www.dcsg.com.au). The membership is a mix of donors and people who have used or may use donor sperm or eggs or embryos, including some adults who were donor conceived. It is an excellent resource.
- Andrology Australia (www.andrologyaustralia.com.au). A brilliant website that has information about reproductive health that every man should know. Director Professor Rob McLachlan is a leading force in Australian andrology and one of the most thoughtful, knowledgeable and pragmatic doctors you could ever meet. In Australia he is my go-to andrologist if I have questions.
- IVF Australia (www.ivf.com.au). My own IVF unit, with an excellent website. It is part of Virtus Health (www.virtushealth.com.au), Australia's the largest fertility provider.
- The Fertility Centre, Wollongong (www.thefertilitycentre.com.au). The Fertility Centre is the low-cost part of Virtus Health. Reducing

costs per IVF cycle allows more access for patients within a large world-class infertility company.

- Facilitator Ruth Pellow (www.ivftreatmentabroad.com). Ruth's unit helps patients find an IVF unit abroad. She links the couple with a European IVF unit for egg donation, sperm or even to use their own eggs and sperm. I only use this unit for Australian couples seeking mostly egg donation and Ruth facilitates the entire experience, including travel, accommodation and medications.
- Dr Janet Hall (www.drjanethall.com). Janet has written many book and articles about sex that you are sure to find useful.
- Dr Rosie King (drrosieking.com.au). A sex therapist.

New Zealand

- Fertility New Zealand (www.fertilitynz.org.nz). The national network for those seeking support and information in New Zealand on fertility issues.

United States

- American Society for Reproductive Medicine (www.asrm.org). The ASRM annual meeting, attended by nearly 10,000 fertility-related experts, is one of two in the world I regularly attend. ASRM has excellent guidelines for patients.
- RESOLVE: The National Infertility Association (www.resolve.org).A non-profit charitable organisation to help men and women with infertility.
- American Fertility Association (www.theafa.org). Another leading American group.
- Centers for Disease Control and Prevention (www.cdc.org/repro-ductivehealth/infertility). Cover issues of reproductive health and infertility.
- American College of Obstetricians and Gynaecologists (www.acog.org). Has a lot of fact sheets.
- Reproductive Facts (www.reproductivefacts.org). The direct ASRM patient facts website has facts by leading health professional and is extremely reliable. with excellent information.

United Kingdom

- Human Fertilisation and Embryology Authority (www.hfea.gov.uk). This organisation can help you choose a British IVF unit.
- British Infertility Counselling Association (www.bica.net). Offers information to patients seeking details of counsellors specialising in infertility.
- National Institute for Health and Care Excellence (www.nice.org.uk). Provides guidelines on infertility.
- www.gettingpregnant.co.uk. If you're thinking about getting pregnant go to this is an excellent website, which covers lots of infertility issues.
- Fertility Network UK (www.fertilitynetworkuk.org). A national charity for those with fertility problems.
- Endometriosis UK (www.endometriosis-uk.org). A national endometriosis group.
- Adoption UK (www.adoptionuk.org). You can also look at www.adoptionregister.org.uk, the British Association for Adoption and Fostering (www.baaf.org.uk) or the Intercountry Adoption centre (www.icacentre.org.uk).

Europe

- European Society of Human Reproduction and Embryology (www.eshre.eu). The pre-eminent European organisation. I regularly attend their annual conference, along with 10,000 other delegates.

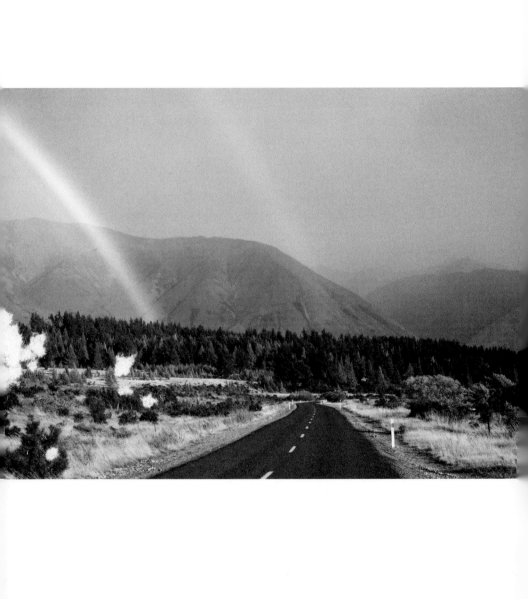

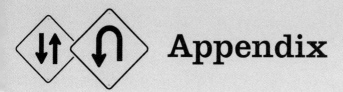

Appendix

Abstract delivered by Dr David Greening at the 25th annual meeting of
the European Society of Human Reproduction And Embryology,
Amsterdam, 28 June – 1 July 2009

'**K**eep the river flowing': An exploratory study to assess the effect of daily ejaculation for 7 days on semen parameters and sperm DNA damage.

 ## Introduction

The optimal ejaculatory frequency for human fertility is yet to be determined. This study assessed semen quality after daily ejaculation for seven days as compared to a standard three-day abstinence period. We hypothesised that frequent ejaculation (FE) may be a physiological mechanism to reduce sperm DNA damage while enabling standard, WHO-defined semen parameters to stay within the normal, and presumed fertile, range.

 ## Materials and methods

One hundred and eighteen men with a history of infertility, recurrent miscarriage or repeated IVF failure, were enrolled based on evidence of elevated sperm DNA damage as determined by the sperm chromatin structural assay (SCSA). This assesses sperm DNA integrity based on the percentage of sperm with a high susceptibility to low pH-induced DNA denaturation, and is expressed as the DNA Fragmentation Index (DFI per cent). The entry criterion was a DFI >15 per cent. After three days of abstinence, semen parameters were assessed by strict WHO criteria.

Men were then instructed to ejaculate daily for seven days with re-assessment on day seven. No other treatments or lifestyle change interventions were offered. All one hundred and eighteen men completed the seven days of ejaculation.

Results

	After three days' abstinence	After seven daily ejaculations	Confidence interval difference	Significance (paired t-test)
Count (million)	183.8	70.9	84.4 – 142.1	P < 0.0001
Concentration (mil/ml)	61.7	43.6	11.4 – 25.4	P < 0.0001
Volume (ml)	3.5	2.0	1.3 – 1.8	P < 0.0001
Rapidly progressive motility	27.2%	31.8%	-7.6 – 1.7	P < 0.005
Slowly progressive motility	14.5%	14.5%	1.6 – 1.8	n.s.
Total motile (including non-progressive)	49.0%	54.1%	2.2 – 7.8	P < 0.001
Non-motile	7.3%	7.7%	-1.5 – 0.6	n.s.
Normal morphology (strict)	2.2%	2.5%	-0.6 – 0.2	n.s.
DFI	33.9%	25.8%	5.9 – 10.4	P < 0.0001

Ninety-six men (81.4 per cent) exhibited a decrease in DFI (mean decrease 12.1 per cent), whereas twenty-two men (18.6 per cent) had an increase in DFI (mean increase 9.6 per cent). Frequent ejaculation significantly decreased semen volume and sperm density, without compromising sperm motility, which rose slightly but significantly. While there was no change in morphology on very strict WHO criteria, the changes in DFI were substantial in degree and statistically highly significant.

Conclusions

There is no evidence-based consensus about ejaculatory frequency in advising couples attempting to conceive. What is known is that intercourse on the day of ovulation offers the highest fecundity rate. But what is the best advice leading up to ovulation or to egg retrieval for IVF?

Previous studies have shown that increased periods of abstinence are associated with sperm DNA damage. We have previously shown that increased ejaculatory frequency can reduce sperm DNA damage, we believe by reduced exposure to reactive oxygen species in the testicular ducts and epididymis through forcing a faster transit time. This could account for the improvement in DNA seen in 80 per cent of the men. The remainder who had an increase in DFI might have a different explanation for their sperm DNA damage not amenable to the present remedy, perhaps a process leading to apoptosis or to a defect in protamination. We observe that ejaculation frequency also has no obviously beneficial effect on the proportion of immotile sperm.

This present study involved ejaculating daily for seven days. The optimal number of days of ejaculation might be more or less than seven days but a week appears manageable and favourable. It seems safe to conclude that couples with relatively normal semen parameters should have sex daily for *up to* a week before the ovulation date. In the context of assisted reproduction this simple treatment may assist in improving sperm quality and ultimately achieving a pregnancy.

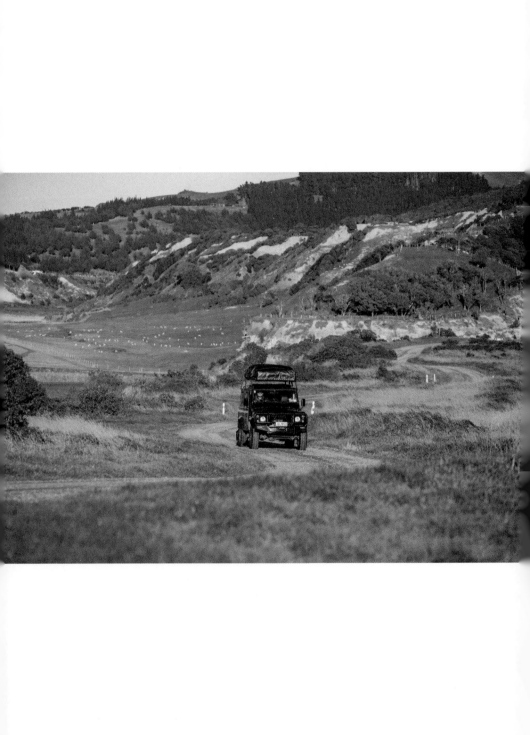

Acknowledgements

Writing a book is a journey all of its own; you travel a road that only you really know. Along the way you meet many helpful people.

My grateful thanks go to my wife, Sian, who has been patiently behind me throughout the many years it took me to finish this project.

Gary, who wrote the foreword, was the inspiration for the book. When he and Sue sat in my office in Sydney in 2003 I had little idea of what would come to pass.

I asked the routine question about IVF: 'How many IVF cycles have you done?' They replied: 'Thirty-two'. I thought I'd misheard them and said, 'Pardon?' I hadn't.

I suspected Gary had high sperm DNA damage hidden in his otherwise very normal semen analysis results. I was considering using donor sperm when I had a light-bulb moment on O'Connell Street, Sydney – apologies to the pedestrian who bumped into me when I stopped suddenly. The story is in the book.

Talking later to Gary (he is now the father of two children) about his ten-year journey through IVF, I came to realise he had travelled with Sue but was otherwise totally alone. Gary is a nice guy, quiet and unassuming, yet when I phoned and asked him about this time he got really upset. Never once in ten years did a single person ask Gary how he was; it was always about Sue.

I presented my study of one hundred and eighteen wonderful men with high sperm DNA damage like Gary at a conference in Amsterdam. It got world attention and a reporter said to me that I should write a book for men, as there were none. Another light-bulb moment!

My sincere and grateful thanks to Australian author Hazel Flynn, my wonderful mentor. She has guided me along the literary road that all novice writers travel. I have benefited greatly from Hazel's experience; she knows the world of writing like doctors know the world of medicine. Countless texts, emails and phone calls later I could tell her I had a publisher.

Staff at my practice have helped greatly. Sheree, my practice manager, turned each manuscript submission into the perfect form each publisher wanted in her perfectionist way.

My thanks to the prominent Melbourne sex therapist Dr Janet Hall, who worked with me on the sex chapter. It was a privilege to work with her.

Bill Twyman had the first job of editing and condensing the original manuscript. Hazel informed me that no author can easily cut down their own book and strongly suggested I get an editor.

I asked friends and relatives to read chapters and offer suggestions. My brother Mark, himself a published author, gave advice when asked. Many kind couples reviewed it over the years and colleagues like Dr Rob McGrath offered their opinions.

Thank you to all who contributed to the writing of my book. If I don't acknowledge you directly, thank you all the same! You know who you are.

To my publishers **Rockpool Publishing**, thank you for taking on *A Road Map to Fertility*. There were many rejections from publishers before I got a phone call from **Lisa Hanrahan** and her amazing team to say they wanted to publish my book. Lisa 'got' the concept of a book written to engage the male partner. She has enormous enthusiasm as a publisher and a person; you need that as an author. The green light to publish, however, is just the start of the process, and Lisa and Rockpool guided me through the long journey to the destination. It is somewhat like arriving at the edge of a city after a long drive, then negotiating through the city until finally you reach the end. In some ways the complex driving parts are in those final kilometres, and that's when publishers show their worth.

Writing a book is a journey; when it is finally written you feel a real sense of achievement. I want to thank my own book for the opportunity to delve into a world you only read about, the world of someone writing a book. I really enjoyed it.

They say that everyone has a book inside them; maybe so. I have thoroughly enjoyed the journey of writing; the experience has been so worthwhile. If there is a book inside you, take it out for a drive and see where it goes.

To you, the readers, I thank you for reading my book. I sincerely hope it helps guide you on your own journey towards becoming a parent.

Index

implantation of 14, 106
sex of 24
transfer numbers of 181
endocrine disease 97
endometriosis 49, 105-7, 110, 111, 124, 138, 143
endometrium 26, 31, 34, 110
environment 76-7, 96, 121, 149, 159
epididymis 16, 18, 37, 122
epilepsy 106
erectile dysfunction 67
erections 8, 9, 90-1
estrogen *see* oestrogen
Evenson, Donald 41
exercise 73

F
facilitators, reproductive 202-3
fallopian tubes 2, 101, 107-9
    ectopic pregnancy in 108-9
    pelvic inflammatory disease in 108
    structure of 27-8
    tests of 140
family history 121, 125
fecundity 81
females
    age of 81-6, 102, 123, 148
    alcohol consumption in 72-3, 125
    anatomy of 101-2
    brains of 101, 102
    conception in 123
    family history of 125
    gynaecological symptoms of 124
    health history of 122-5
    infertility causes in 101-14
    medication use 125
    menstruation in 124; *see also* menstruation
    Pap smears for 125; *see also* Pap smears
    pregnancy in 123
    puberty in 24-5, 102
    recreation of 125
    reproductive parts of 23-34
    sexual frequency in 124

surgery in 124
weight of 157-60
Femara 161
fertility; *see also* infertility
    abstinence 74
    age as a factor 65-6, 79-90
    alcohol 72-3
    chemotherapy 75
    drugs 71-2
    environment 76
    exercise 73
    factors affecting 22, 63-77
    failed treatments 190-3
    heat 73-4
    medications 74
    obesity 66-7
    preconception health 75-6
    radiotherapy 75
    smoking 69-71
    timing for 2
    underweight 69
fibroids 109, 163
fimbria 27-8
follicle 25, 31, 180
follicle-stimulating hormone (FSH) 21, 24, 31, 102, 132, 137, 161-2, 174, 175, 176
follicular tracking 52
fostering 196
free radicals 41
freezing
    eggs 185, 186
    embryos 113, 172-3
    sperm 154, 185
Frick, Francis 36
FSH *see* follicle-stimulating hormone

G
general practitioners 115-16
genes 101
genetic blueprint 7-8, 14-15
genetics 4, 7-8, 36, 39
    aging and 81-6
    disorders in 92-5
    female 81-6